How Can We Talk About That?

Overcoming Personal Hang-Ups So We Can Teach Kids the Right Stuff About Sex and Morality

Jane DiVita Woody, Ph.D., M.S.W.

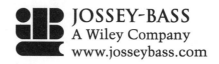

JOSSEY-BASS
A Wiley Company
www.josseybass.com

Published by

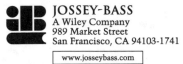 **JOSSEY-BASS**
A Wiley Company
989 Market Street
San Francisco, CA 94103-1741

www.josseybass.com

Jossey-Bass books and products are available through most bookstores. To contact Jossey-Bass directly, call (888) 378-2537, fax to (800) 605-2665, or visit our Web site at www.josseybass.com.

Substantial discounts on bulk quantities of Jossey-Bass books are available to corporations, professional associations, and other organizations. For details and discount information, contact the special sales department at Jossey-Bass.

We at Jossey-Bass strive to use the most environmentally sensitive paper stocks available to us. Our publications are printed on acid-free recycled stock whenever possible, and our paper always meets or exceeds minimum GPO and EPA requirements.

Library of Congress Cataloging-in-Publication Data

Woody, Jane DiVita.
    How can we talk about that?: overcoming personal hang-ups so we can teach kids the right stuff about sex and morality / Jane DiVita Woody.— 1st ed.
        p. cm.
    Includes bibliographical references and index.
    ISBN 0–7879–5914–6
    1. Sex instruction. 2. Sexual ethics. 3. Parent and child. 4. Parenting. I. Title.
    HQ57 .W67 2001
    649'.65—dc21   2001003955

FIRST EDITION
PB Printing   10 9 8 7 6 5 4 3 2 1

Contents

In memory of my parents, Benny and Josephine DiVita

*Dedicated to my husband, Robert Henley Woody,
and our adult children, Matt, Bob, and Jennifer*

Foreword

Whether as a function of shyness, conventional inhibitions, embarrassment, past sexual issues, or current problems, parents today generally have a difficult time speaking with their children about sex and sexuality. Probably it wasn't talked about much, if at all, at home when they were growing up, nor was much additional assistance provided by the programs they were exposed to as children. As a result, the first information children receive about sex typically does not come from their parents.

To remedy this situation, several major issues must be addressed. First of all, parents must be assisted in their efforts to break the pattern of silence, to overcome whatever hang-ups prevent them from speaking, and to learn how to communicate effectively with children regardless of their age. Parents then must have access both to information about sex and to effective techniques for sharing this information in meaningful ways with their children. And such an approach must also be able to fit in with their moral, spiritual, and religious values and beliefs. Ideally, parents should be provided with the tools to educate their children about sex in a positive manner, one that honors their personal values and encourages thoughtfulness, respect, and appropriate sexual behavior.

Successfully dealing with this complex combination of issues requires guidance from a person with a unique combination of knowledge and sensitivity, and Jane DiVita Woody is the ideal candidate for the job. She brings to this formidable challenge the wisdom gathered from many years of experience as a sex education teacher, a trainer of sex educators, a researcher, a social worker, a family therapist, and a parent. By harnessing her skill for engaging writing and speaking clearly and understandably to a broad audience, she has written a book that is truly significant in several ways.

In Part One, she gives parents ideas and suggestions that help them to understand themselves more fully so they can move beyond their personal resistance to focus on the task of speaking with their children about sex. In subsequent chapters she offers a format for sex education that encourages parents to work together to educate their children at various ages and stages of development. Through the use of interactive activities such as role-playing and other exercises, Woody provides parents with a step-by-step program for working through their personal issues so they can practice *before* they preach. She also gives constant attention to the dynamics among family members and to their various backgrounds and the potentially different kinds of experience each may bring to the discussion. Perhaps most striking, she not only acknowledges and respects the importance of moral and spiritual values and beliefs relative to sex education, but offers suggestions that are open to personal interpretation from a wide variety of perspectives as well.

Much has been written about the need to improve sex education, but generally the focus is on programs developed through the schools. Little attention has been given to helping parents in their efforts to become effective sex educators for their children. *How Can We Talk About* That? helps parents feel empowered to handle this challenge and learn ways to take responsibility for teaching their children about sex and sexuality.

Dorothy S. Becvar, Ph.D.
President and CEO of The Haelan Centers
St. Louis, Missouri

Preface

Several years ago, while on sabbatical from the university, I was in Tallahassee, Florida, preparing to write a book on sexuality. The thrust of the book wasn't clear at first until one day when I read a letter to the editor of the local newspaper—suddenly a light bulb went on in my head and I knew that I had to focus on parents as sex educators for their children.

For several consecutive days, the newspaper had been reporting a dispute in mediation between two city police officers, male and female. The two had allegedly engaged in sex while on the job—in a cemetery. The male officer had been fired, and rumors surfaced that he had had the female officer get on her hands and knees and, during the course of a sexual interlude, made her bark like a dog. Confronted with this account, the male officer insisted that she had taken the initiative: she had unzipped his pants and begun performing the act, and he didn't remember how far it went. This testimony led to the next day's headline labeling him a "wronged man."

The story didn't end there, however. That same day, a mother wrote to the editor asking for help in explaining to her twelve- and fourteen-year-old daughters the meaning of the dog-barking, cemetery-sex story. She suggested that given the example set by adults, it was no wonder that children were out of control and had lost respect for their elders.[1] This mother found herself in the impossible situation of having to be a sex educator and moral guide for her children and being unprepared for the job. She was probably thinking, How can I explain these sexual behaviors? I'm not even sure I understand them. How can I explain the irresponsibility of these adults? Their immorality? Police are supposed to be role models. What facts about sex should I pass on to my kids? What do I tell them about right and wrong and how to behave in regard to sex? How do I do all this when I'm so angry, disgusted, and confused?

The Tallahassee story pales in comparison to the media coverage of subsequent sex scandals among public officials and celebrities, especially the Clinton-Lewinsky affair and subsequent impeachment proceedings. Parents and commentators alike, outraged by the X-rated content on the evening news, wondered how to shield youth from the sordid details and hoped to escape questions about oral sex and semen on clothing. Emotions were palpable: clearly the public preferred that sex talk between parents and children be kept to a minimum and be left to parents' private discretion. It wasn't fair that these public sexual revelations had usurped the parental right to *avoid* sexual discussions.

I began to take heart from the media coverage of these sexual escapades: parents might actually benefit from a kick in the pants that would force them to discuss sexual matters in family talks. But parents' complaints about the prospect meant that they truly needed help—a lot of help. Because of my clinical experience over two decades in providing individual, marital, and sex therapy to many clients and teaching a graduate course in sexuality, I had an idea about the kind of help that might make a difference. It was simple: parents need to first resolve their own personal hang-ups before they can take a conscious and active role in their child's sexual and moral education. Even though the idea is simple and logical, the task itself is forbidding.

Another part of my strong commitment to this idea has personal roots. I knew that if I could learn to talk about sex with my husband and children and also to teach and counsel people about it, then anyone can learn to become more comfortable in parent-child sexual discussions. Growing up in a Catholic family with an over-protective Sicilian father, I received a big dose of moral values and principles and almost no sexual information. And at that time, the lessons I did receive, plus the love and support my family showered on me, served me well. I knew the rules and lived by them, as did most other girls in my town.

Still, all the rules and taboos did not stop my curiosity about sex or my eagerness to learn. Boccaccio's *Decameron*, Ovid's *Art of Love*, and other classic and contemporary novels unbelievably found their way into our immigrant home and into my adolescent hands. The excessive strictness I lived with didn't negate girlhood romantic fantasies, crushes, and longings. And it didn't keep me from exploring my own body and sexual response. But I definitely could have used some information and discussion to explain why my eleven-year-old girlfriend was raped, why our neighbor stood nude in front of the window of his house as kids made their daily trek to and from school, and why a local woman always dressed in men's clothing. Eventually I learned all this and much more on my own. But today it's far too risky to leave children ignorant of sexual facts when everything around them pushes them to learn on their own—from friends, the media, or trial-and-error experience.

These pages express other personal convictions. The first one is that I, like most parents, wish that I had done a better job with my own children's sex education. Looking back, I am satisfied with a lot of things: the books we read together when they were young, my consciously calm demeanor in certain situations, my insistence that they take the school sex education courses when available, my willingness to answer questions honestly, my respect for their privacy and offering books with comprehensive sex information, even into their college years. But I regret that we didn't talk more about the complexity of intimate sexual relationships, that I didn't ask about or respond more to their personal lives, and that I didn't tune into more opportunities for these talks.

Another personal motivation is my interest in understanding, uncovering, and dismantling the powerful emotions and beliefs that keep parents more or less on the sidelines of their children's sex education. We watch the plays and moves, we worry, but we never quite get into the game ourselves. Even with the best of intentions and the desire to foster our children's sexual health and moral soundness, we often simply cannot break from the family history, past learning, and personality characteristics that make us hesitate and hold back. This unconscious reluctance is extreme for some parents, and I have wanted to better understand and address this topic for a long time.

Read on to discover ways to confront and conquer whatever hang-ups, big or small, might keep you wary of your child's sexual questions and concerns. Out of this endeavor, you can move toward a proactive rather than a reactive position and play a major role in fostering your child's positive sexual and moral development.

Jane DiVita Woody
Omaha, Nebraska

Author's Note

All of the clinical case vignettes and other anecdotes referred to in this book derive from my counseling, research, and teaching over several decades and typify concerns common to many people. To protect individuals' privacy and anonymity, I have changed names and details so that these stories represent composites and literary constructions. Any similarity of these names and stories to actual known individuals is purely coincidental.

Acknowledgments

Many people have contributed encouragement, suggestions, and technical assistance that helped make this book a reality. I am deeply grateful for their interest in the idea and their faith in my ability to finish the project.

First, I want to thank my editor, Alan Rinzler, first for listening, understanding, and supporting the central idea behind the book. Once the project was under way, his superb editorial guidance and dedication enabled me to produce the finished product and meet deadlines.

Special thanks go to my colleagues at the University of Nebraska at Omaha, especially the College of Public Affairs and Community, which awarded me a sabbatical to get started on this project. Henry D'Souza and Robin Russel, my coinvestigators for the adolescent study mentioned in the book, also played a part in helping my ideas germinate. Henry and another colleague, Amanda Randall, also worked with me on a study dealing with mothers as sex educators for their children. I am grateful for the help provided by several graduate student assistants: Brett Phillips, Carol Hardy, Maggie Milner, and Brad Hove. Joyce Carson's expertise in word processing was a godsend as she helped me, in the final stages, put the manuscript into consistent computer files and formats. Throughout the years, too many students to name have reacted positively to my ideas about parents and sex education and often shared their own experiences and stories, all of which helped clarify my approach to this book.

Beyond my workplace, there were others who supported this book in various ways. My dear friends and colleagues Jean Regester, Mary Springer, and Deborah Silver labored through early versions or excerpts and gave me valuable comments and suggestions. Father Robert Pagliari also carefully reviewed a recent version of the book and offered useful editorial guidance. Harvey Hester, a colleague in AASECT, meticulously read the previous version of the manuscript and offered both encouragement and thoughtful suggestions for style and content.

Finally, I am most appreciative of the energy and attention that my husband, Robert Woody, gave as he read more versions of this book than I care to acknowledge. His comments and suggestions were always on target and insightful. He also showed understanding and patience as much of my life became focused on deadlines and hours sitting at the word processor.

J.D.W.

Introduction

I had always heard that you wait until your kids ask about sex and then you answer their questions. That's what I was prepared to do. The only thing is my boys are fourteen and sixteen; they never asked, and I don't think they will now.

Talking with kids about sex, answering their questions, keeping them from self-destructing over loves gained and lost—none of this has ever been easy. But now young people face a crisis they didn't create: every day, their current and future sexual health is at stake. But most of us parents just don't get it! We're still procrastinating or pussyfooting around with the facts of life and love, leaving our sex-crazed culture in charge of bringing up the kids. And many of us never ask, *Why am I so scared of this job?*

This book answers that question. After years of research, field work, counseling, and collective experience, I have concluded that personal hang-ups are behind most of our anxiety. The greatest obstacle to providing sexual health for the next generation is our own attitude. That's why it's up to us, the grown-ups, to get over our issues and unresolved conflicts about sex so that we can provide better guidance and inspiration to our children. This book offers a plan to do exactly that. Now, by working through the first three chapters in sequence, you can learn to overcome these hang-ups and give your children a better sex education and greater hope for sexual health than we ever got.

Have you talked with your teen about sexual intercourse (or even said the word to him or her), its risks, and your values with regard to it? Have you mentioned that over two million teens a year contract a sexually transmitted disease? Have you told your son what to expect at puberty? Do you let your preteen daughter dress in sexy styles but leave her uninformed about her sexual organs?

Even if you have had a talk, or even several, you are still not finished. Like most people, you probably contend with a rush of feelings—embarrassment, irritation, anxiety. Maybe you try to talk, but the words don't come out right. Or you cut the conversation short. Or you say, "Go ask your mother [or father]."

These uncomfortable feelings and reactions of inertia, avoidance, and procrastination connect to issues in your own life. The purpose of this book is to show you what to do about them. I believe that once you face and overcome your personal hang-ups, you can then get on with the business of teaching your child the right stuff about sex and morality. And don't worry—this doesn't mean talking to your kids about your sex life! In this case, as in many others, good boundaries between parents and children remain important. Rather, it means taking an honest look at yourself—past and present—and coming to terms with what you find.

- Did I make sexual mistakes as a young person?

- Do I want my child to do it differently?

- Do I now have a good sexual relationship with a loving partner?

- Am I clear on my beliefs about sex and morality, for myself? For my child?

These are just a few of the questions that parents don't want to think about. But getting answers is the key to being straight with kids about the facts of life in a way that will keep them listening. Most parents want to achieve this goal and are willing to figure out why they are so emotional about their kids' sexual concerns and questions. In the past, sex experts have discounted parents' emotional reactions and offered simplistic advice: take a more disinterested approach toward sex, learn the facts about sex, talk to your kids about sex in spite of your discomfort and embarrassment. But until now, no one has ever suggested that parents' ambivalence about sex is what renders them dumbfounded or paralyzed by their children's coming of age, and parents need more than simple platitudes to get beyond that.

This book supplies the missing piece to the puzzle of why parents bail out even when youngsters face the sexual perils of today's culture. Overcoming your hang-ups will help you figure out what you want teach your kids about sex and morality and free you up to learn how to do it well.

Modern life has created sexual risks for young people that were unimaginable a decade ago. Unfortunately, most of our kids face these issues alone or with the "help" of their friends. The reason: many parents remain unable or unwilling to teach their kids sexual survival skills for the twenty-first century. Too often, even today, the major approach to family-based sex education is "Don't ask, don't tell." And our society and culture, instead of offering meaningful help to change this pattern, are a big part of the problem. The offerings of the media and politicians have the effect of keeping sexual preoccupation high but sexual ignorance and confusion even higher. Although many parents would like to give their kids a better sex education than they themselves had, they don't know how, primarily because they haven't a clue as to why they avoid or bypass this aspect of parenting.

Now, for the first time, a real solution is at hand, and it isn't merely to latch on to buzzwords like *abstinence* or *safer sex*. This book guides you through the steps to becoming a credible sex educator and moral guide for your child. In taking on the mission to foster sexual health for the next generation, you gain two added benefits: you can improve your own sex life and contribute to the overall sexual health of our society.

Kids in Crisis

Today the sexual health of young people in the United States and in most industrialized countries in the world is at risk. Conditions in modern society propel children toward sexual decisions and behaviors that can harm their physical and mental health and leave lifelong scars. The media, the changing structure of family life, and the new teen culture push kids to grow up fast and take on adult behaviors, including sexual relationships, before they are ready in mind, body, heart, and spirit. Parents need to take a critical yet clear-eyed look at the confusing and dangerous environment young people face every day.

Brave New World

There are great advantages to being alive at the dawn of the twenty-first century, but the complexity of this age calls for new skills to cope with how this changed world affects sexuality. Sexual messages of every shape and form constantly tantalize and promise sweet rewards. So-called mature adults struggle every day with sexual issues that bring them or their families much misery—affairs, unwanted pregnancy, obsession with pornography, compulsive sexual behavior, and criminal sexual acts. If adults succumb without quite knowing what hit them, how much more vulnerable are youth in this same environment?

Through every media venue, children are constantly exposed to sexual images, messages, topics, and innuendo. The parents who cringe at the thought of their child asking about a high-profile sex scandal apparently remain unaware that children already have daily access to a steady diet of sensational, demeaning, trivial, superficial, stereotyped, and overly romantic notions about sexuality. Because these messages are packaged to have a strong emotional appeal, they influence at the unconscious level and begin to permeate and define the child's sexual self. From movies, videos, music videos, computer games, the Internet, cable television, television sitcoms, soap operas, and "trash" talk shows, the themes are so common they are often hardly noticed. For example:

- Sex is for the young, thin, and beautiful.

- Sexual success defines human happiness.

- Sex is romantic and spontaneous.

- Sex means being out of control, even bizarre, sometimes brutal.

- Peculiar, kinky, or aberrant sexual behavior is entertaining.

- The ideal female partner is a sex-crazed nymphomaniac.

- The ideal male partner is a stud.

- Having a loving relationship defines a woman's identity and self-esteem.

- Making sexual conquests defines a man's identity and self-esteem.

How do these qualities figure in your definition of a morally sound and sexually healthy child (or adult, for that matter)? Unless this fast-food approach to sex is counterbalanced by a good, strong dose of the facts about the pleasures, complications, and moral implications of sexuality, young people are at risk of ending up with a distorted, if not disordered, sense of sexual identity. But the media rarely offer informational discussions about birth control, AIDS, sexually transmitted diseases (STDs), or other important sexual topics that might correct or neutralize the media blasts of "myth-information." So if you aren't teaching your kids what is factual, real, and meaningful about sex, just think about what is filling the vacuum in your child's soul.

Media Effects

Recent research studies have begun to document the influence of the media. One study showed that in television and film portrayals of women being killed, in 25 to 30 percent of cases there is a sexual overtone (in the shower, making love, undressing). Another study showed that males, after viewing an R-rated movie, had less sympathy and empathy for the victim shown in an enactment of a rape trial than a control group that viewed nonviolent material.[1] Do you ever think of how these images could deaden your young son's sensitivities or dominate his masturbation fantasies?

The Internet too has truly ushered in a new world. Given the fascination that people have with sex, it is not surprising that the word *sex* is the number one topic for Web searches.[2] Kids don't even have to go looking for sex on the Web; they readily encounter unsolicited pornography, with much of it coming through e-mail chat rooms where they think they are talking with other children.[3] One source predicts that by 2002, "close to 50% of children under 12 will be on-line, including about 30% of children under five."[4] At this point, to access thousands of graphic sex sites, children need only say with the click of a mouse that they are eighteen and not offended by adult material.

It is not simply the media's messages and images about sex or life in general that are troubling. It is their pervasiveness and their power. Pop culture and consumerism are dramatically but insidiously defining the identities of adults and children and our notions of the good life. Overworked, overextended, and ambivalent about moral values, many parents seem unable to give their children undivided attention and really get to know their children as people. Instead, they allow the second family of pop culture, the mass media, and peers to mold their children's identities and souls.[5] Parents need to decide whether they will allow this second family to raise their kids or counter it by taking charge of their family. Adults who themselves oversubscribe to the cults of youth and consumerism can hardly protect their children from the culture's sexual stereotypes.

Growing Up Fast and Loose

Other elements of today's world compound the usual sexual risks, driving youth toward poor sexual choices or limiting their ability to choose. Drugs are available in all communities, and young people, including college students, accept and use alcohol as a routine part of social life. In addition, youth violence and gang life often promote early sexual activity as a status symbol and even sexual crimes as an initiation rite. Although the greatest risk falls on boys and girls who live in the midst of violence and other chaotic life conditions, many so-called privileged youth also encounter the culture that links teen violence to drugs. Both spill over to affect sexuality in many ways.

Middle-class adults like to think that youth violence has geographical or socioeconomic boundaries. But that's a myth. Violence and drugs, which have "influenced the youth culture to an incalculable degree," are not only present in poor inner-city locations but also have penetrated suburban and rural neighborhoods and schools and the various media that transmit pop culture.[6]

Consider also other sociocultural changes: greater personal freedom for both young males and females, less family time and supervision, less involvement with extended family and neighbors, more experience of parental divorce for many youth, widespread prevalence of overextended single-parent families, and the increasingly wide gap between high-income and poor families. Before they are ready, many children who feel alone and lonely are left to manage complex emotions on their own. It is no wonder that they begin to pursue their own "adult" solutions, such as making their own decisions, rejecting parental limits, and engaging in sexual relationships. These aspects of modern life are part of your child's world, regardless of whether or not they describe your particular family situation.

The Youth Culture

Besides struggling with societal and family upheaval, children, especially teens, also inhabit an exciting, enticing youth culture. Here sex is a primary topic of conversation—who's going together; who's doing it, who's not; who's a fox, a stud, a slut, a tease, a queer, a lesbo, and so on. As early as elementary school, children already hold stereotyped ideas of what qualities make a woman or man attractive or successful. For example, research has shown that eight- and nine-year-old girls often say they are on a diet. A recent study sponsored by the American Psychological Association solicited questions from boys and girls, ages eleven to nineteen. Some of their most common concerns reflected gender stereotypes and sexual issues. Why are girls moody? Why are boys so immature? Why are boys afraid to show emotions? They also asked, however, for sexual information and how to deal with peer pressure.[7]

One message that beams through loud and clear from society and the youth culture is that sex is a big deal—"go for it." And if you honestly recall your own youth, you know that the teenage body and psyche are attuned to follow that kind of impulse. In fact, the trend in the past thirty years is that youth are experiencing sexual intercourse at younger and younger ages, and therein lie the greatest risks. Youth face situations that call for decisions about sex at younger ages than their parents imagine. Yet parents routinely underestimate their teen's involvement in sexual activity.[8]

At the same time, another, perhaps more disturbing, notion in the youth culture is that sex is no big deal. Many teenagers, having absorbed hundreds of hours of sitcom sexual escapades, attach no special meaning to sexual intercourse beyond that of a pastime or game. One teen couple explained to a Planned Parenthood educator what their guidelines were in deciding to have intercourse. He said, "It would be OK if she was willing." She said, "It would be OK if he would go out with me." So sex is what two people do when they are attracted to each other, are dating, are in a steady relationship, are seeking status, or are merely curious. If young people get their initiation into sex with this mentality, then we have reason to worry about their future sexual lives.

The dark, frightening underbelly of the youth culture comes to mind when one hears of a recent horrific murder of a teenaged girl in a small town in Nebraska. The eighteen-year-old boy who committed this crime believed that the girl was pregnant with his child, a situation that didn't fit his plans. Fellow students had talked about their dating as a mismatch; the girl was described as serious and active in school service and the boy labeled the partying type. Rumors abounded but facts were few. It was said that she had told him she was pregnant, but the autopsy indicated there was no evidence of pregnancy in the past three months. Motives, facts, and rumors were never clarified because the boy and a younger teenage boy who was an accomplice agreed to guilty pleas. Regardless, the effects of this tragedy will remain, for the family who lost a daughter, the two boys awaiting prison sentences, their families, and the community that may never heal from these losses.[9]

Out of the Mouths of Babes

Not every sexual mistake brings such tragedy, but teens encounter and take sexual risks every day, all the while feeling unprepared to manage the complicated situations and feelings that their actions bring. Although they want adult or parental guidance, they rarely ask for it, plunging ahead into sexual situations with a trial-and-error approach that's a sure formula for problems. Listen to this recent firsthand account from a group of 129 teens across Pennsylvania. In small focus groups, they explained how sex works in their world, all the risks sex entails, and their thoughts on these matters.[10] Here's what they told us.

1. There is not a lot of communication in male-female relation-ships. Partners don't talk about boundaries, sexual behaviors liked or disliked, or protection. Boys think girls should set boundaries, for the reason that boys often care more about "scoring" and that they, unlike girls, are not stigmatized for having multiple partners.

2. Abstinence can mean various things to teens: waiting until marriage for intercourse, waiting until engagement, waiting for emo-tional maturity and financial responsibility, doing anything other than intercourse, doing anything without penetration, and so on.

3. Decision making about contraception is not a rational process. Teens assume that parental silence on this topic means dis-approval of its use. Other barriers are embarrassment, lack of plan-ning for sex, lack of a driver's license to get to a clinic, worry about a partner's reaction, the expectation that girls should take care of birth control, and no communication between partners. A major factor is that a lot of sexual experiences (they estimate 50 to 75 per-cent) occur not within a relationship but during parties with alco-hol involved or as one-night stands.

4. High-risk sexual behaviors include sex without protection, multiple partners, not knowing partners well, and forced sex. Among situations conducive to these risks are parties that often include alcohol, drugs, and increased peer pressure to engage in sex, and being alone at home with a partner.

5. Body is a big concern; girls feel great pressure to be thin, and both boys and girls are burdened by the need to look or dress a cer-tain way. Very few in the group liked and accepted their bodies.

6. Media images distort sex, and repetitive messages can influ-ence people, but this group thought that these things happen to younger teens and to other people, not themselves.

7. Sexual orientation should not be a basis for judging people. But these teens' lack of knowledge of same-sex orientation was obvi-ous, as they were surprised to learn that gays and lesbians, in strug-gling with their identity, sometimes date opposite-sex partners, marry, and have children.

8. Good sexual decision making calls for good communication between partners, but this rarely happens. These teens had varied thoughts on readiness for intercourse: partners are monogamous and use protection; they love each other; both are ready; both trust and care about each other; both are able to talk about sex; both are able to be seen naked without embarrassment. Finally, they expressed some doubt and cynicism about how sex fits into a relationship, especially a long-term relationship.

9. Neither school nor parents provide meaningful sex education. These teens saw school programs as a "joke," inadequate, irrelevant, "too little, too late." They agreed that parents are most likely to preach, to just tell them not to have sex, and "to think you're doing it" if you ask questions or want to talk about it. They want parents to listen, take the first step, be more understanding, talk about sex from when the child is young, and have many talks.

The thoughts and behaviors of these young people confirm the immediate risks to their present and future sexual health. Sexual activity involving alcohol, drugs, peer pressure, and lack of ability to use protection multiply the usual perils of teenage sexual activity: pregnancy, STDs, coerced or forced sex, loss of self-esteem, and loss of personal and purposeful life goals. Unfortunately, even though they recognize the dangers, many young people see no better alternative than going ahead with sex under these conditions and taking their chances.

Parents in Denial

Just like teens, parents know very well that sexual risks loom large on the horizon of childhood development and adolescent life, yet they often remain unbelievably silent on the topic and even avoid ready-made opportunities to broach the subject. It's as if parenthood automatically confers on adults the right to forget their own sexual history and to deny children's sexuality.

At an intellectual level, we see the need for more parent-child talks, but we don't see ourselves taking the lead or learning how to do this; instead, we wish for an easy solution. Now, however, it's time for a real solution, and the first step is to honestly face the reasons—the hang-ups—behind our inertia.

Parents' Silence and Avoidance

Research studies show that too many parents skimp on their children's sex education and never get around to offering the information and guidance that youth need and want. For many years and continuing today, teens have reported that they learned little about sex from their parents. For girls, mothers may discuss menstruation and the process of conception; and if they give further information, they prefer to talk about sexual intercourse, sexual morality, and birth control. A large majority of both parents and teens (80 percent) agreed that parents never mentioned masturbation, even though these parents thought that children masturbate. In another study, most parents believed that children should be reassured that masturbation is normal (only 16 percent disagreed).[11]

Even when it comes to other issues that pose big risks, such as STDs, HIV-AIDS, and alcohol and drugs in relation to sex, parents don't offer information or strategies for protection. Other topics that go unmentioned are abortion, girls' sexual desire and sexual pleasure, sex in the media, sex-role stereotypes, differences in boys' and girls' reactions to sex, and noncoital sexual activity. Predictably, parents and adolescents often disagree on the amount and content of their discussions about sex. In one study, for example, whereas 75 percent of mothers said they had taught their sons something about sex, only 33 percent of sons reported this.[12]

Parents are not only often silent on most sexual matters but also absent, especially fathers, when others attempt to offer life-saving information about sexual risks. A few years ago in Chico, California, three thousand parents were invited to preview a forty-five-minute AIDS awareness drama before their children in grades nine through twelve viewed it. Only thirty-nine parents attended.[13] What were those absent parents thinking? That AIDS won't touch their children's lives? That they would be uncomfortable or embarrassed to see this topic presented? That teaching about AIDS is strictly the school's business, not theirs?

Given that the specter of sexual risk does not spur parents into talks that might protect their kids, we can be fairly certain that they are not sharing messages about the positive aspects of sex—that is the ultimate taboo topic. Young people know that sex is a great thing, but they are left to sort out the reasons for this by themselves. What makes for good sex? What does sex do for an intimate relationship? What does sex have to do with love? How does sex differ from infatuation, and how does sex change over a person's lifetime? Kids quickly realize that sex, love, and relationships are puzzling but also powerfully rewarding. Yet parents avoid the topic of sexual excitement and pleasure like the plague. They cannot find ways to acknowledge the positive dimensions of sex because they fear that any honesty about its joys and rewards gives permission for sexual activity.

Parents' Helplessness

In spite of the worry about the sexual culture that engulfs their children, most parents don't plan for their child's sex education or initiate it; instead they adopt a wait-and-see attitude and hope for the best. Here's what some of them have told me:

> "It is so hard to deal with this subject. My little girl came up and asked me the other day about her cousin who lives with a man, wanting to know if they were having sex. It just threw me for a loop."

> "My fourteen-year-old daughter is going on her first date this weekend, and I'm worried already."

> "My eight-year-old granddaughter has started asking me about sex. I told her to ask her mother, but I don't think her mother has told her anything."

When asked, parents say that they do want their children to learn about many aspects of sexuality, and they realize the need for earlier, better, and more parent-child talks about sex. Yet they continue to back away from taking the initiative to make these talks happen. In research studies, young people say that their parents need sex education to help them communicate with their kids better;[14] however, parents look to a different solution. Recently, 97 percent of parents in a large study wanted school education programs to teach children how to talk with parents about sex and relationships.[15] This notion seems a desperate cry for help from parents who see themselves as incapable of learning to do something that is so complex and stressful.

The "Can't" Checklist

The aforementioned report tells us what we already know in our hearts: talking to children about sex is difficult—so hard that parents *want schools to teach their children how to approach parents on sexual matters!* What kind of thinking or reasoning accompanies this kind of helplessness? Let's take a quick inventory. Do you shy away from, avoid, cut short, postpone, or feel overwhelmed at the prospect of giving your child sexual information and moral guidance? Reasons for these responses may be mostly unconscious, and you can't consciously deal with something you are not even aware of. See if any of the reasons on this list strikes a nerve for you.

- I'd feel funny using the correct names of the genitals.

- I'll explain everything when we have our "talk."

- I don't know enough about sex myself.

- I'm too embarrassed or uncomfortable about sex.

- My child will be embarrassed to hear me talk about sex.

- I don't know how much to tell my child or when.

- I might end up looking ignorant or stupid.

- I don't want to trigger my child's curiosity or interest in sex.

- I just want to tell my child about the dangers—"don't do it."

- If I tell my child about protection, this is a mixed message or permission.

- I'm afraid my child will ask about my sex life—past or present.

- My sex life is a mess, so how can I help my child?

Once you become aware of your reasons—what holds you back— you can begin to face them in the light of day and evaluate them.

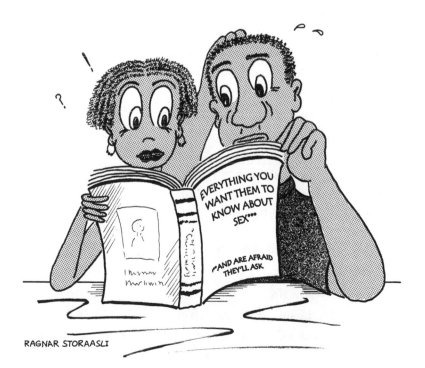

RAGNAR STORAASLI

Although this book urges you to change yourself—not to wait for the schools to change your kids—parents and families are only part of the problem. Real and lasting change can come only from understanding all the forces invested in keeping things the same.

Why the Problem Has Persisted

Who would have thought that so many members of the baby boom generation would fail with their kids' sex education—just as their own parents did? We have to look to several factors to understand why rational talk about sexuality is still so rare at the dawn of the twenty-first century. In the past decade, pockets of resistance to school-based sex education have intensified into a highly vocal and polarized debate about family values—the so-called culture wars between so-called social conservatives and progressives. Although the public in general has consistently supported school-based sex education programs, and parents today want these to be comprehensive, the will of the majority is not in place. Public school and other government programs now predominantly reflect the restrictive ideology of abstinence-based sex education supported by only a vocal minority of our population.

This social and political atmosphere has added to parents' own confusion about their child's sex education. Should we, can we, in good conscience, teach our children abstinence? Or safer sex and protection? If not, then what should we teach? Our ambivalence connects to confusing, perhaps painful, memories or images of our own sexual history and life.

Resistance to Sex Education

A great many events and new developments in the world are calling for a change in how we guide youth toward a healthy sexual identity and a meaningful future. Yet the winds of change have encountered tremendous resistance from an opposite direction. A vociferous minority demands a halt to open, factual discussions about sexuality and calls for a return to the "traditional" moral code of the "good old days." These are often the same critics who blame every social ill on "sex education," whether offered by schools or parents.

Followers of this formula intentionally and incorrectly equate sex education with sexual permissiveness in order to devalue it. And no political or cultural happening passes without demonizing sex education (or feminism or the sexual revolution) as the villain. Following Monica Lewinsky's interviews on publication of her book, the conservative columnists appearing on the editorial pages of major newspapers attributed her behavior and demeanor to sex education—not to her personality, genetic heritage, family structure, parenting, sexual exploitation by a teacher, exposure to pop culture, or other potential influences—only to sex education. For example, commenting on Lewinsky's television interview with Barbara Walters, Mona Charen wrote: "Sex educators of the world, take a bow. Monica and millions like her have absorbed your message. Sex is shorn of moral dimensions or considerations. It is the greatest achievement to be 'comfortable with [one's] sensuality.' "[16]

How do you react when you hear social critics (representing only a minority of Americans) denounce comprehensive sex education? Research studies have always shown wide public support for sex education in the schools. And today the majority of parents want the schools to teach more, not less, about a variety of sexual topics, including *both* waiting to have sex *and* condom usage. A recent study found big gaps between what parents wish would be discussed in school sex education classes and what is actually covered, according to students. Parents' wishes and students' reports agree that many schools are teaching the core elements of sexual risk, HIV-AIDS, other STDs, and the basics of pregnancy and birth. But as for other information, the study found that it is sorely missing. Maybe you, like the majority of those parents, want classes to cover more, such as the following topics:[17]

- Waiting to have sex

- Birth control

- Abortion

- Homosexuality and sexual orientation—that is, being gay, lesbian, or bisexual

- How to deal with pressure to have sex

- How to deal with emotional issues and consequences of being sexually active

- How to get tested for HIV-AIDS and other STDs

- How to use condoms

- How to talk with parents about sex and relationship issues

- How to use other birth control methods and where to get them

- What to do if you or a friend has been raped or sexually assaulted

- How to talk with a partner about birth control and STDs

If you want your child to have comprehensive sex education, the bottom line is that you will need to make it happen. Once you learn to overcome the hang-ups, you will be able to talk about these topics with your child as well as lobby for the schools to do a better job.

The Culture Wars, School Sex Education, and the Government

It is no accident that comprehensive sex education in the schools doesn't take place at the level that parents desire. The battle over sex education has been at the center of the culture wars for over a decade, and the traditional, restrictive sexual ideology has come to dominate public school sex education programs. Many programs have chosen not only to include abstinence as a part of sex education programs but also to omit critical sexual information, discussion of psychological factors, and communication skills, all of which are relevant to sexual risks.

The dominant restrictive ideology holds that schools, including public schools, should focus on influencing young people not to engage in sex; consequently, comprehensive information about sexuality is seen as likely to increase sexual activity and thus as incongruent with the goal. Although research has not supported this connection between information and activity, "just say no" abstinence-based education has taken center stage. The result is sex education programs that compromise basic democratic ideals. That is, public schools in a democracy should provide full information about sexuality and acknowledge that diverse religious and ethical sexual ideologies freely exist in a pluralistic society; they should not promulgate any one ideology. This kind of curriculum would enable students to learn firsthand the democratic ideals of freedom of inquiry, critical deliberation, and freedom of belief.[18]

The Federal Government's Policy on Abstinence Education

Governmental agencies have obviously played a part in installing the present restrictive ideology in the sex education enterprise, but their role has been that of responding or acquiescing to what is essentially a vocal minority (when you consider the list of sexual topics that many parents want the schools to teach). The proponents have not only the ear of the federal government but also its rubber stamp. The Welfare Reform Act of 1996, which automatically renews in 2001, awards abstinence education funds to states as part of the welfare reform effort. To qualify, projects must offer programs and use materials that comply with the definition of abstinence education contained in the 1996 act. The eight-point definition "became law without the benefit of public input or Congressional debate. The language that created welfare reform abstinence education was inserted into the legislation 'during a process that is reserved for corrections and technical revisions.' "[19]

Most people would agree that delaying sexual activity is a good choice for young people. And for anxious and tongue-tied parents, the idea of teaching abstinence may seem like a worry-free solution: "If you don't do it, you won't be at risk." But the definition in the 1996 act has larger implications for sexual health, both in the short run and the long run, for young people and for adults.

Parents need to think about all of the eight points in the definition of abstinence education, because several raise legitimate questions about medical accuracy, defining sexual activity, setting marriage as the standard and only outlet for sexual activity, and restricting information. An overall concern is whether the strictness of the definition, which reflects a single moral view of human sexuality, conflicts with the establishment of religion clause of the U.S. Constitution.

 ## Personal Inventory

Response to the Federal Policy on Abstinence Education

Directions. With the goal of learning something about yourself, consider the following components of abstinence education, which have been quoted from the 1996 act.[20] Take inventory as to whether you endorse these concepts about abstinence, whether you want this as a framework for giving your kids the "right stuff" about sex and morality, and whether you want public schools to teach only these principles as the basis for sexual health. My additions (bracketed and in italic type) following each component in the definition bring up related issues to think about. After reading and thinking, place your response on the line in front of each item: a plus sign (+) if you agree or a minus sign (–) if you disagree with the item on abstinence education.

Abstinence education means an educational or motivational program that

_____ 1. Has as its exclusive purpose, teaching the social, psychological and health gains to be realized by abstaining from sexual activity [*not to include other information that may promote protection against sexual risks; not to define sexual activity*]

_____ 2. Teaches abstinence from sexual activity outside marriage as the expected standard for all school age children [*assumes that marriage is the only outlet for sexual activity*]

_____ 3. Teaches that abstinence from sexual activity is the only certain way to avoid out-of-wedlock pregnancy, sexually transmitted diseases, and other associated health problems [*does not acknowledge that research shows higher failure rates for abstinence than for other birth control methods*]

_____ 4. Teaches that a mutually faithful monogamous relationship in the context of marriage is the expected standard of human sexual activity [*assumes that only monogamous heterosexual marriage embodies the purpose of adolescent and adult human sexuality*]

_____ 5. Teaches that sexual activity outside of marriage is likely to have harmful psychological and physical effects [*does not acknowledge research that does not support this very broad statement*]

_____ 6. Teaches that bearing children out-of-wedlock is likely to have harmful consequences for the child, the child's parents and society [*does not acknowledge many other factors besides pregnancy outside of marriage that might affect consequences*]

_____ 7. Teaches young people how to reject sexual advances and how alcohol and drug use increases vulnerability to sexual advances [*may lack impact if overall program lacks credibility because, for example, it assumes that marriage is the only avenue for sexual expression*]

_____ 8. Teaches the importance of attaining self-sufficiency before engaging in sexual activity [*does not define sexual activity; does not*

*provide a standard of self-sufficiency that acknowledges
sexual activity among people who marry young or who lose
self-sufficiency during marriage for various reasons, such as
loss of job, health, and so on]*

What did you learn from your responses to this inventory?

- Are you clearer on your beliefs about abstinence?

- Are you more aware of the need to talk more openly
  and repeatedly with your child about sexual activity,
  relationships, risks, and ways to promote sexual health?

- Are you more thoughtful of ways to present your beliefs
  and values about sex to your child at different ages and
  stages of development?

- Are you more committed to learning from your child
  what he or she hears about sex and abstinence at
  school and from others outside the family?

- Are you more convinced of the greater importance of
  your role as a parent than that of the schools in your
  child's sex education and moral guidance?

- Are you more determined to lobby for the kind of sex
  education that you value for your community?

All of these are desirable outcomes.

It's unfortunate that sex education programs are now offering less
sexual information at the very moment that the culture and media
intensify the obsession with sensational, trivial, unrealistic, and com-
mercialized portrayals, uses, and abuses of sexuality. The quality of
school programs and the debate over sex education are two reasons
why we must worry about the sexual health of the younger generation. These social factors intensify parents' personal concerns about

sex (and they already have plenty of these), leaving them feeling helpless to influence their child's sexual understanding and decisions.

Boomers Befuddled

As several recent scholarly books have noted, the cultural upheaval of the sexual revolution, along with its ideals, gains, and excesses, gave way to the conservatism of the counterrevolution and the drawing of battle lines for today's culture wars.[21] Parents of the baby boom generation have experienced both forces in their own sexual lives, and now many haven't a clue about how to foster their child's healthy sexual development.

Both the sexual revolution and counterrevolution have a lot to do with parents' failure as sex educators and moral guides for their children. Because of the sexual revolution, many adults during the past thirty years became more free and uninhibited about sex, and they thought these were good qualities. For example, they may have accepted nonmarital sex as a private matter between consenting adults and freely engaged in this behavior. They may have also believed that removing ignorance and shame about sexuality was a good value that could be passed on to children. They may have imagined it was possible to approach human sexuality with some degree of rationality and inquiry. But somewhere between young adulthood and parenthood, the ideals of factual sexual information and honest, rational dialogue died out for many baby boomers.

Although the increasing negative social commentary on the sexual revolution may have triggered personal doubts, adults rarely changed their own sexual behaviors. And even with the increasing rates of sexually transmitted diseases and the HIV-AIDS threat, people have not reverted to sexual repression and inhibition. Instead they have become resigned to living with "their own moral contradictions and intellectual inconsistencies."[22] An accurate observation of this phenomenon was the comment made by Dr. Georgia Witkin, a psychologist who appears on television talk shows: "Men want their daughters to abstain, but not their girlfriends."[23]

Some of us may never think about our personal sexual behavior and moral beliefs until we face the prospect of our children's emerging sexuality. And if this brings our buried contradictions to the surface, we quickly push them down, knowing how hard it would be to expose personal doubts to the kids. At this point, internal conflict takes over, and for many reasons. Perhaps we cannot reconcile our own permissive sexual behavior with the sexual guidelines we want to pass on to our children. Maybe our own past or current sexual behavior has brought problems, regrets, and disappointment that now haunt our psyches. Flooded with feelings of embarrassment,

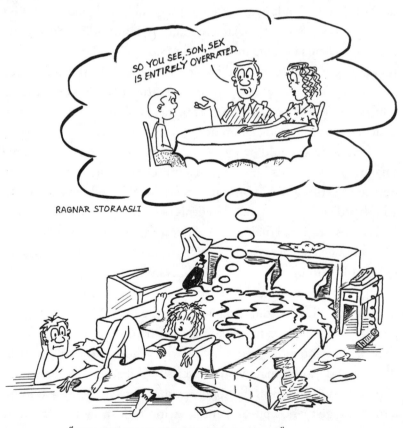

RAGNAR STORAASLI

"EVER FEEL LIKE WE'RE BEING HYPOCRITES?"

ignorance, confusion, worry, guilt, or shame, we understandably avoid children's sexual questions or situations.

Clearly, many seemingly well adjusted adults remain ambivalent about human sexuality. Although they may act on their sexual desire and enjoy sexual pleasure, they have never rationally and consciously arrived at a set of sexual values and standards of conduct that they truly believe in and follow. They may not experience their sexual lives as wholesome, satisfying, and meaningful. Without this sense of congruence, partners rarely talk thoughtfully and honestly to each other about sex. Without this sense of congruence, parents remain doubtful and anxious about their sexuality and thus destined to feel like ignorant or shameful children. Without a congruent adult sexual identity, they can hardly give clear messages to children about sexual facts, relationships, and morality.

An Invitation and the Promise of This Book

The younger generation has not created the crisis in sexual health, and young people are not the only ones with sexual troubles. Sexual hang-ups affect both parents and the larger society. Because many parents feel uncertain, even ashamed, about their own sexuality and sex lives, they dance around their child's sexual concerns or muddle through with few or no facts and a lot of warnings. And their children carry on the same legacy when they become parents. Society, which can only reflect the deep ambivalence of its members, plays its part in the vicious cycle of sexual ignorance and confusion.

In this book I invite you to make a change that can make a difference—in your own private life, in your child's life, and in the life of society. My message in this book is that parents must take center stage in their child's sex education. You have the responsibility not only to act in this family drama but also to produce and direct it. Simply furnishing a script, such as the facts of sexuality or a set of questions and canned answers, is not the goal of this book. This method would not remove the hesitance and mixed messages that result from ambivalence about your own sex life and confusion about the sexualized world in which today's children live.

Begin your journey through this book by completing the chapters in Part One sequentially. Personal preparation through taking inventory, doing your own thinking, and overcoming hang-ups is the real formula for success. By working through this book, you can find meaningful answers to the challenges that human sexuality poses for us in both youth and adulthood. With effort and courage, you can change your own sex life for the better, help your child achieve both sexual health and moral responsibility, and halt the generational legacy of silence and shame about sexuality that creates personal and social problems.

Part I

Overcoming Your Sexual Hang-Ups

1

Taking a Personal Inventory for Moms

You say you love; but then your hand
No soft squeeze for squeeze returneth,
It is like a statue's—dead—
While mine to passion burneth—
John Keats, "You Say You Love"

Of course, dads and other men are welcome to read this chapter, but I want to address specifically the mothers, grandmothers, aunts, and other women who may be involved in raising our next generation. We know there is a difference in being female, not only in our sexuality but also in how we've been brought up, conditioned by society, treated in the media, and considered by society at large.

These experiences become hardwired into our psyche and play out in everyday life. We don't choose to feel dissatisfied with our sex life or anxious about our child's sexuality, but we often end up with these unwanted outcomes anyway. Rather than attempt to understand causes, we cart out rationalizations—that sex is just too complicated or that it's vastly overrated. After all, what can we expect from growing up in families and a society that provided little sexual information and lots of mixed messages?

Now is the time to break with timidity and quiet desperation. It's possible to openly face and overcome your hang-ups. Making this change will not only help you feel better about yourself but can also free you to become a credible sex educator and moral guide for your child.

This chapter invites you to take inventory of your sex life. Whether you are married, divorced, or single—whether you are with or without a partner—you have a sex life. It encompasses several dimensions of your identity, both past and present: your sense of being a woman; your feelings and thoughts about your appearance, attractiveness, and personality; the kind of partner you desire; your sexual knowledge, attitudes, and values; and your experience, feelings, and thoughts in regard to love and sexual relationships.

Taking inventory means taking the pulse of your sex life and deciding whether it is alive and well or weak and sickly. This is an opportunity for self-discovery, and I believe you will find it intriguing and rewarding. As you gain new insight and make changes if they are needed, you become stronger for the task of guiding your child toward sexual health.

Sexual hang-ups come in big and small sizes. But they all seem to affect our ability to think of our kids as sexual beings and to help them survive the risks of growing up. Through the years I have heard mothers casually make comments that reflect apprehension about this aspect of parenting.

> "I can handle telling my six-year-old daughter how babies grow and develop, but I just can't imagine letting her know that her daddy and I 'did it' to bring her into the world."

> "My fifteen-year-old son has become such a good-looking young man, and I know the girls are going to start calling him. I just don't even want to think about it."

> "Things are so different today. At my daughter's school they hear all about abstinence. When I was growing up it was all about sexual freedom."

If you have ever had thoughts like these, treat them as a signal that some sexual hang-up is haunting the depths of your psyche. Tune in to find out what's behind the worry. Unresolved memories or past experiences can be part of a current and continuing uneasiness about sexuality. Consider the following questions to see whether anything in your history might be triggering a sexual hang-up.

- Did you engage in sexual activity as a child or teen, alone or with partners?

- With partners, what were your motives and what were your reactions?

- Did you take risks (using no protection, using alcohol or drugs, having multiple partners)?

- Did you ever experience an STD, pregnancy, abortion, or have a child out of wedlock?

- Were you ever molested, coerced into sex, or sexually assaulted?

- Did you avoid sex or love relationships because of personal choice, fear, feelings of inadequacy, or lack of opportunity?

- How do you evaluate your previous serious love or sexual relationships (satisfying, meaningful, disappointing, hurtful, shameful, and so on)?

- Have you made an effort to learn about human sexuality and better understand in what ways accurate sexual information can benefit your sex life?

What were your feelings as you reviewed these questions? Paying attention to your emotions and putting a name to them is the first step in defining your hang-ups. When people contemplate their sex lives, their initial emotional reactions tend to mirror their most honest thoughts and judgments. Perhaps you felt mostly comfortable when you answered the questions. If your first feelings weren't obviously positive or negative but veered instead toward worry, ambivalence, or confusion, you may have been trying to avoid even more uncomfortable emotions. If you immediately felt a rush of anger, shame, dread, hurt, disgust, or despair, take these intense emotions a sign that you have some current hang-ups to deal with.

Emotions: The Pulse of Sexual Life

A child whose parents enjoy a happy sex life is lucky indeed. Their positive feeling about sexuality has a good chance of translating into a comfortable, competent approach to their child's sex education. When a sexual issue comes up, they are more likely to think about it rationally, rather than have their intellectual ability "shorted out" by a lightning bolt of painful emotions. Parents who have sexual hang-ups can expect their underlying worrisome or painful feelings to surface unpredictably in the face of almost any sexual topic. As the following scenario shows, merely *talking* about sex education (not actually doing it) produced a highly charged emotional reaction that led to avoidance, withdrawal, anger, and blame.

Several years ago, Dan, a graduate student in my course called Analysis and Treatment of Sexual Problems, recounted a troubling conversation he had had with his wife Dell. This was the gist of it.

DELL: Dan, you left the book for your sex class just lying on the table in the family room. You ought to think about the kids and watch where you leave it.

DAN: You think it would hurt the kids if they saw it?

DELL: Well, they're just kids. They don't need to see that kind of book.

DAN: Did you look at it?

DELL: No, why would I?

DAN: You might learn a thing or two.

DELL: I thought this was about the kids.

DAN: It is, and I don't think that learning about sex is a bad thing. Susie is eight and Danny is ten. Have you told them any of the facts of life?

DELL: Have you? They're too young.

DAN: I saw Susie watching that Danielle Steel movie with you. She was really taking in all that kissing and groping. They already know more than you think.

DELL: You just have a filthy mind.

DAN: At least, I can enjoy sex. But I had to work at it.

DELL: You mean that's all you think about.

DAN: Look, Dell, let's get back to the kids. I don't want Danny to go through what I did.

DELL: What was that?

DAN: I was eleven. First time I had a wet dream it scared the hell out of me. I thought I was sick. I couldn't ask anyone. I didn't know anything or how to find out anything.

DELL: Well, you go ahead and talk to Danny if you want. When Susie is older, I'll tell her what she needs to know.

Strong but unacknowledged emotions permeate this conversation. Dell is embarrassed by the book on sexuality and uncomfortable with the idea of giving the children sexual information. Part of her reaction seems linked to her feelings of anger and disgust toward Dan's sexuality, which imply dissatisfaction with her husband's approach to sex and with her own sex life. Dan's comments too reveal an underlying irritation with his wife's anxiety about sex. Without changing her view on the children's sex education, Dell abruptly ends the conversation and refuses to team up with her husband to deal with this matter.

Rather than ignore or deny the feelings that sexual topics trigger, you need to identify them and the message they hold. Several interesting exercises lie ahead as part of your preparation. These will help you think further about your sex life, become aware of your emotions about it, evaluate its quality, and consider how it might affect your approach to your child's sex education. In addition to gaining personal insight, you will also need to take action. If you uncover inhibitions, concerns, or serious problems, you will learn to resolve these in ways that allow you to enrich your own sex life and start guiding your child toward sexual health.

Women and Stereotypes of Female Sexuality

I believe that a major contributor to women's sexual hang-ups is the social programming they receive when they are growing up. Although many of us have swallowed some of the culture's stereotypes about female sexuality hook, line, and sinker, as adults we don't have to let them continue to dictate our behavior. Exactly how does our culture define female sexuality and the roles expected of women? Think in terms of the dos and don'ts, such as, "Girls shouldn't date around too much" or "Women should let their partner take the lead in sex." We have all sensed, heard, and tried to live by rules like these and many more—whether or not they felt right for us.

Before exploring how rigid gender roles can produce unhealthy attitudes toward sex and wreak havoc on women's sex lives, take a minute to complete the following brief inventory and learn or relearn something about yourself.

Personal Inventory

Level of Sexual Pleasure

Directions. Answer the following questions, keeping in mind your marital relationship or, if you aren't married, your current committed relationship or, if you aren't in a committed relationship, your most recent ongoing sexual relationship. Place your answer in column A. Later you will come back and add an answer in column B.

	A	B
1. How many times during a typical, average day do you have a pleasurable sexual thought, fantasy, image, or genital sensation?	____	____
2. How many times during the course of a typical month do you experience sexual desire or interest on your own (not in response to your partner's desire)?	____	____
3. How many times during the course of that typical month do you act on your own desire by initiating sexual activity with your partner, in a very direct way, verbally or physically?	____	____
4. How often do you typically experience orgasm when you engage in sexual activity with your partner? Rate on the following scale: 0 = 0%, 1 = 25%, 2 = 50%, 3 = 75%, 4 = 100% of the time when engaging in sex.	____	____
5. Would you like to experience orgasm more often? (0 = no, 1 = yes)	____	____
6. Have you ever clearly told or shown your partner the kinds of touch, caress, activity, or stimulation that you enjoy or that bring you the most pleasure or to orgasm? (0 = no, 1 = yes)	____	____

	A	B

7. How many times in the past six months did you masturbate and reach orgasm alone?   _____ _____

8. Rate the physical and sensual gratification you derive from sexual activity in a typical sexual encounter with your partner. (0 = none, 1 = a little, 2 = some, 3 = a lot, 4 = completely satisfied)   _____ _____

9. Rate the psychological and emotional satisfaction you derive from sexual activity in a typical sexual encounter with your partner. (0 = none, 1 = a little, 2 = some, 3 = a lot, 4 = completely satisfied)   _____ _____

10. Do you have a favorite image, scenario, memory, or fantasy that you see as an ideal or exciting sexual encounter? If yes, close your eyes and imagine this for a minute. What are the exact ingredients? (See the note in the text on how to score this item.)   _____ _____

Now go back to each item, and in column B rate the amount of anxiety or embarrassment and discomfort that you experienced in answering each item. Use the following scale: 0 = none, 1 = a little, 2 = some, 3 = quite a bit, 4 = a great deal.

Scoring. Here is how to score question 10. If you had no ideal sexual scenario, score 0. If you did, go back to your ideal sexual scenario, decide which one of the following is the major ingredient, and score accordingly. If your imagined fantasy focuses on your own physical desire, physical arousal, or genital excitement or pleasure, or focuses on pleasurable physical, sexual acts involving your or your partner's genitals, score 4; if kissing and nongenital touching and caressing are the focus, score 3; if holding, talking, or both are the focus, score 2; if a romantic setting, activity, or ambiance (for example, music, candlelight, beach, dancing, clothing) is the focus, score 1.

Now add all the numbers on the lines in column A to arrive at your total item score. Next, add all the numbers in column B, which rates your anxiety, to arrive at your anxiety score. You can enter these scores here:

_____ Total item score

_____ Anxiety/embarrassment/discomfort score

Interpreting your scores. This inventory is highly focused on only a few aspects of your sexuality. It is not an indicator of your overall satisfaction with your sexual or intimate relationship. So, that said, what can it tell you?

The *total item score* reflects your level of sexual desire, the degree to which you are motivated to act on it, and the value you place on physical and sensual sexual pleasure. Are you satisfied with your level of desire? If so, are you satisfied with your frequency of acting on it? If not, is it something about you or the relationship or your lifestyle that keeps you from initiating sexual activity? Are you satisfied with the level of physical pleasure that you receive from your sexual encounters? The lowest possible score is 0, which suggests a total disinterest or disavowal of sexual desire and pleasure. Another negative scoring pattern consists of high numbers on sexual desire and interest (questions 1, 2, and 5) but low numbers for acting on or achieving sexual pleasure (questions 3, 4, 6, 7, and 8). On these five items, the higher numbers mean that you take greater initiative to experience sexual pleasure and that you derive physical satisfaction from your sexual activity.

The *anxiety score* reflects the amount of negative emotion that you feel about your level of sexual desire and the physical pleasures of sex. Is your anxiety high for the questions about independent sexual desire? Is your anxiety high for the questions about the pursuit of pleasure (masturbation, orgasm, physical gratification)? A total score between 0 and 10 suggests very little negative emotion; 11 to 20 suggests some; 21 to 30 suggests quite a bit; and 31 to 40 suggests a great deal of negative emotion. The idea here is to *reflect* on what these numbers mean for you. Do they cause you to think about your sexuality in a different way? Do they enable you to face some personal concerns that you typically ignore or avoid? In the next section, we continue to explore how understanding stereotypes about female sexuality can help you identify and overcome sexual hang-ups.

Society's Double Standard

In many ways, society endorses male sexual desire and need for pleasure as a normal, innate pursuit. In contrast, women's sexual interest and need for pleasure have been minimized and marginalized. Women can be "horny" and sexually turned on as long as this is *in response to* a husband or male partner with whom they have a loving relationship. And even when a male partner gives an eager female partner permission to fully enjoy sexual pleasure, in other contexts (the locker room, breakup of the relationship, refusal of sex, and so on) he may slap a disparaging label on her (slut, whore, tease, lesbian, and the like). This kind of experience, and other forms of it, can leave women and girls ambivalent about or alienated from their sexuality. As a result, they may get little enjoyment from sex, inhibit their erotic interests, or simply devalue the notion of sexual expression, even with a loving partner.[1]

What are we to make of the findings of a nonscientific Ann Landers survey in 1985, in which 72 percent of the ninety thousand women responding said they would be content to be held tenderly and forget about "the act"? Of the women giving this response, 40 percent were under the age of forty.[2] How would a mother who views sex in this way present sexual information to a daughter or to a son? Did these women ever enjoy the sexual act? If so, when, and why did they cease to find pleasure in it? Simple surveys never answer the really important questions. But here you can find your own answers, discover what they mean, and move on to solutions if needed.

Ambivalence About Female
Sexual Desire and Sexual Pleasure

In addition to constant exposure to society's negative stereotypes, there are other reasons why women feel ambivalent about sexual desire and sexual pleasure. This response could have roots in a fairly typical adolescent and family life, or it could stem from traumatic sexual experiences ranging from sexual pressure or coercion to rape or other forms of childhood or adult sexual abuse or assault. Clearly, sexual trauma, especially if repeated or never resolved, is likely to have the most serious impact. For some women, traumatic sexual experiences can result in such extreme anxiety, shame, and disgust with sexual activity as to produce various types of sexual dysfunction, as well as other mental health problems. The next section addresses these more serious sexual problems, but here we will briefly consider the more typical ambivalence about sexual pleasure that is common to many women who have no history of sexual trauma.

My clinical work over more than two decades brought me into contact with numerous women who were uncertain about their right to sexual pleasure or who did not take ownership of their sexuality. Some clients openly admitted that they wanted to have better sexual functioning to benefit their husbands, not themselves. Women with perfectly normal female bodies saw themselves as not measuring up to some ideal female body image. It's no wonder that during sex their energy centered on concealing their perceived flaws rather than on having a satisfying, pleasurable experience.

Anna, a thirty-four-year-old married mother of two children, captured these attitudes in her written response to a body awareness exercise that I assigned her to do at home—looking at her nude body in a mirror. "The top half from my waist up is disproportionate with the bottom half. In relation to my buttocks which stick out so far, I guess my tummy does seem flat. I also have saddlebags and thick thighs. . . . If my fifteen-hundred-plus miles jogging [through the years] turned out to be preventative inches, I'd hate to see what

I would look like if I hadn't taken up the exercise. . . . Now I'm not thrilled about wearing shorts everywhere in summer except they are cooler. I wonder why Steve does not object to seeing me in short shorts like I do."

Another young woman, Beth, entered therapy because she and her husband were considering having a child and she worried whether their marriage would last, given her intense dislike and avoidance of sex. Beth clearly said that she was not interested in changing for herself but wanted to improve their relationship. She too recorded a litany of body flaws: "sagging breasts, flabby thighs and knees, cellulite on the back of my legs, and my hips really look wide when I'm sitting down."

The problems and attitudes of Anna and Beth stemmed from various causes, including personality, stresses in the family of origin, dissatisfaction with their partners, and lack of sexual information. Nonetheless, some of their attitudes are quite pervasive in our culture and affect women who never seek therapy and never resolve negative or ambivalent feelings about their own sexuality.

As already mentioned, society barely acknowledges that females do or should experience sexual desire. Today, in spite of the sexual revolution and more openness about sex, women are still seen as primarily interested in a loving relationship. A common expectation is that they express sexual desire more as a romantic rather than physical need, or that they primarily feel sexual interest in response to a male partner's sexual desire. Girls growing up today are not likely to have many experiences that would contradict these attitudes. Many messages about sex warn them about males' persistent pursuit of sex, with the implication that girls' own sexual interest is too inconsequential to mention.

Few girls ever hear from any source that their own sexual desire is a normal, healthy, natural response. Those who experience masturbation may discover that they have desire as well as the capacity for sexual pleasure, but the power of social programming often diminishes this knowledge—especially if they judge the behavior as wrong or abnormal. In the case of teenagers having sexual inter-course, the focus is likely to be on the male's, not the female's, sexual pleasure. Thus my study of adolescent sexuality found a huge difference, not unexpected, between the percentage of males (75 percent) and females (18 percent) who reported feeling "sexually satisfied" from their first experience of intercourse.[3]

The Instrumental View of Female Sexuality

Another factor that devalues female sexual desire and interest in sexual pleasure is the apparent energy that girls themselves place on being chosen for a relationship, keeping a relationship, and satisfying a boyfriend's sexual desire. Consequently, when they do engage in sex with a partner, a major motive may be to show their love to the partner or commitment to the relationship, rather than to gratify their own sensual and sexual needs. Here's how one young woman, eighteen-year-old Lindsay, put it: "When you're younger, you're told by your friends that guys are assholes, they're pigs, they're basically just trying to get in someone's pants. And the girls are like, 'I think I'm gonna let him. I'm gonna let him sleep with me.' It's not, 'I'm gonna make love to him.' It's, 'I'm going to let him do this to me,' like a reward or something. If you didn't, you were a tease. And if you did, you were a slut. A lot of adults still think that way."[4]

Considering that society reinforces in various ways the scenario Lindsay describes, women often enter adulthood and marriage with an unconscious instrumental view of their own sexuality. In other words, they may regard it somewhat as a commodity to be exchanged for love or a commitment, rather than as a valued dimension of their own identity and a source of personal pleasure. Once the desired love and commitment seem secure, some women scoff at the continuing importance their male partners place on sex. All too often, women seem willing to bypass sex if their bodies don't meet the "standards" of sexiness or when they get busy with jobs, children, or family life. Hence the results of the previously mentioned Ann Landers survey.

This unconscious retreat from sexual pleasure does not mean that women do not enjoy sex or do not initiate sex at times. The telling response is whether they tune into their own sexual desire and unashamedly allow themselves the physical pleasure. How many women view their sexuality with pride as part of their individual sexual identity, as a normal part of their body and spirit that entitles them to sexual pleasure for themselves and not simply as a gift to satisfy or acquire a partner or to sustain a relationship?

Men and women in relationships struggle to find the common ground that will allow them to enjoy sex. The flip side of the double standard is the similarly restrictive, stereotyped approach to sex that society assigns to men. (See Chapter Two for a complete discussion of the stereotype of hypermasculinity.) As a result, gender battles in the bedroom are common. A typical complaint from men is that women too often refuse their sexual invitations; women protest that men are too aggressive. Clearly, partners whose sex lives suffer from difficulties like these need to find better solutions than to simmer in resentment.

It takes courage and honesty to look at ourselves and determine how much we buy into rigid sex roles, but it takes even more effort to begin to neutralize their power over our lives. Only we can decide the behaviors and expectations that we will truly endorse because they suit us and meet our needs. One guideline is to strive to embrace all dimensions of our sexuality. If we don't, we unconsciously pass on rigid attitudes about both female and male sexuality that could affect the sexual health of the next generation.

Women's Sex Lives

First, let's dispel the myth that the course of anyone's sexual life is a smooth one. The road to becoming a sexual being is typically filled with hills and dales, bumpy roads and detours, and some smooth sailing. As I mentioned before, various characteristics and life experiences can combine to cause sexual difficulties. Left unresolved,

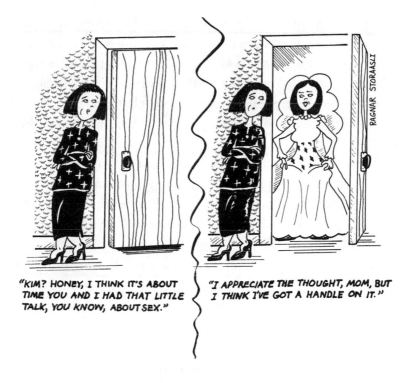

"KIM? HONEY, I THINK IT'S ABOUT TIME YOU AND I HAD THAT LITTLE TALK, YOU KNOW, ABOUT SEX."

"I APPRECIATE THE THOUGHT, MOM, BUT I THINK I'VE GOT A HANDLE ON IT."

these become hang-ups big and small. Whether in or out of our awareness, they tend to deaden our overall sense of happiness and well-being and leave us anxious about teaching our kids about sex.

Thorns Among the Roses

Even when they enjoy sex and have no major problems with desire, arousal, or orgasm, some women may still experience uncomfortable emotions about sex. In these situations, they likely harbor minor sexual dissatisfactions that erupt intermittently to sting and prick. These eruptions are especially likely to occur if a woman's sexual concerns hover out of her awareness, remaining largely unconscious. They can also happen when a woman is aware of the sexual concern but takes no action to resolve it.

If this description fits you, you might have an unwanted intense emotional reaction in an unexpected situation, such as when your partner makes a sexual overture or your child asks a sexual question. This chapter gives you the chance to bring such sexual hang-ups into conscious awareness and consider options to resolve them. (The last section in this chapter offers specific recommendations for resolving these problems, such as by changing attitudes or behavior or by redefining the concerns in a way that defuses their impact.)

Before exploring the more serious sexual and relationship disturbances, let's consider some of women's most common sexual worries. I see these more as irritants that lurk under the surface—but still wear you down—like a splintery thorn in the flesh that goes unnoticed until the skin reddens and pain strikes.

To learn more about yourself, review the following list of less serious sexual concerns that mostly involve your personal sexual identity. (The next inventory covers more serious sexual problems.)

 ## Personal Inventory

Level I Sexual Concerns

Directions. Put an X in front of any item that is a concern you currently experience and a second X on the line if you need to resolve the difficulty. For example, you might need to resolve a problem if it causes negative emotions, thoughts, or behaviors that interfere with your sense of well-being or the kind of intimate and family relationships that you want. Resolving such a difficulty could entail changing behaviors or adopting more rational or balanced thoughts and attitudes, such as letting go of past mistakes or forgiving yourself. Conversely, some of the concerns that you experience may not be sufficiently relevant or distressing to have a negative impact on your current life.

_____ 1. Lack of sex education or sexual knowledge that leaves me feeling ignorant or inadequate

_____ 2. Shyness or timidity in communicating with my partner or child about sexual matters

_____ 3. Past sexual choices and behaviors that I regret or feel guilty about

_____ 4. Dissatisfaction with aspects of my body, features, or overall appearance

_____ 5. Ambivalence about my sexual values

_____ 6. Lack of congruence between my professed sexual values and actual behavior

_____ 7. Uncertainty, as a single mother, about how to handle my dating and intimate relationships in regard to my child

_____ 8. Confusion about the sexual values and moral code I want for my child

_____ 9. Current sexual choices and behaviors that I regret or feel guilty about

_____ 10. Unwanted or excessive sexual inhibitions within my committed relationship

_____ 11. Unresolved shift in my personal sexual values, beliefs, or conduct (for example, from liberal to conservative or vice versa)

_____ 12. Occasional questions about my sexual orientation

_____ 13. Feelings of being devalued or treated unfairly because of being a female

_____ 14. Discomfort, embarrassment with the sensual or physical aspects of sexual pleasure

_____ 15. Concerns about physical, emotional, or sexual reactions due to menstrual symptoms, menopause, or perimenopause

---

At this point, a quick count of the double X's can suggest whether one or more difficulties are keeping you from having a happier sex life. (Later you will return to these when you're ready to take action to resolve them.)

Not surprisingly, these kinds of hang-ups can create an inexplicable wariness about our children's sexuality, as I have seen when conducting groups for mothers that focus on children's sex education.

At age forty-four, Leah is in a happy second marriage and thoroughly enjoying her sex life with her husband. She had grown up with traditional parents who were silent about all sex matters. During her late teens and early adulthood, Leah felt liberated by the attitudes of the sexual revolution and had several satisfying sexual relationships before her first marriage. Though she remembers taking some risks, she had no problems. Now, with her fourteen-year-old daughter, she is reluctant to go beyond the basic information about menstruation and reproduction. After talking this over with several other mothers, she figured out why. She resents all the negative messages about teenage sex that are in the media, but part of her says that maybe abstinence is the best guideline for kids today. She thinks that being sexually active was good for her, but doesn't know what message she wants to give her daughter.

With a different history and for different reasons, Leslie, age forty, has a past that keeps her unconsciously timid and avoiding sexual discussions with her two young adolescent daughters. Leslie's parents had been strict during her teen years and, on occasion, intrusive and accusatory when she began to date. They had not given her any sex education but implied a lot of dangers and warnings about sex. She was a virgin until she met her husband-to-be and was comfortable with the decision to have sex before they were married. Their sex life continues to be very satisfying and exciting. Leslie says she has counted on school programs to give her daughters their sex education. When challenged by other mothers in the group, she recognized that she is reluctant to talk with her daughters because she wants to respect their privacy, she wants to trust them in a way that her own parents didn't

trust her, and she believes that she and their father are
good role models for responsible behavior.

The legacy of their early and current sex lives can affect women's
attitudes toward their own sexuality and that of their children. As
the situations of Leah and Leslie illustrate, inhibitions can be powerful even for women who enjoy sex, and can render them passive
or silent when their children need sex information and moral direction. And for those women who do have personal sexual dissatisfactions, too often they submit to the taboo of not talking about sex
and simply move their sexuality to the bottom of life's priorities.

Big Trouble in Paradise

Serious problems, such as a sexual dysfunction, an unhappy love
relationship, or unwanted sexual behaviors take a toll on women's
overall well-being and intimate relationships. A recent survey on
sex in the United States found that sexual dysfunction, including
desire, arousal, orgasmic, and pain disorders, are more prevalent
among women (43 percent) than among men (31 percent). For
women, elevated risk for these sexual problems is linked to younger
age (eighteen to forty-nine), the experience of sexual trauma, and
single status (never married, separated, divorced, or widowed). Only
about 20 percent of the women reporting sexual dysfunction had
sought professional help for their problems.[5]

Besides dysfunction, other individual sexual and relationship problems create dissonance that can affect your sense of well-being and
satisfaction with your sex life. To learn more about yourself, consider
whether any of the disturbances in the following list trouble you.

Personal Inventory

Level II Sexual Concerns

Directions. Put an X in front of any problem that you currently experience and
another X if you need to resolve the problem. For example, you might need

to resolve a problem if it causes negative emotions, thoughts, or behaviors that interfere with your sense of well-being or the kind of intimate and family relationships that you want. Resolving such a difficulty could entail changing behaviors or adopting more rational or balanced thoughts and attitudes, such as letting go of past mistakes or forgiving yourself. Conversely, some problems that you experience may not be sufficiently relevant or distressing to have much effect on your life situation or choices.

_____ 1. Sexual dysfunction (problem with desire, arousal, or reaching orgasm, or pain during sex) in myself or my partner

_____ 2. Severe overall dissatisfaction in my marriage or committed relationship

_____ 3. Cheating by me or my partner in a relationship based on fidelity

_____ 4. Unresolved childhood or adult sexual trauma for myself or my partner

_____ 5. Incongruence and dissatisfaction with the sexual orientation or gender identity that I or my partner presents to the public

_____ 6. Sexual disorders in myself or partner, such as unwanted sexual fetishes or criminal sexual offending

_____ 7. Problems in adjusting to the loss of my partner through divorce, death, disability, or ending of the relationship

_____ 8. Inability to find or maintain acceptable dating partners or the kind of intimate relationship that I want

_____ 9. Sense of despair or disgust toward all sexual and intimate relationships

_____ 10. Indiscriminate, risky, or compulsive sexual behavior

---

A count of the double X's can suggest whether one or more of these serious difficulties are keeping you from having a happier sex life. (Later you will return to these when you're ready to take action to resolve them.) Having completed the last two inventories, you will likely have a sense of whether you harbor some minor or major sexual hang-ups that deserve your further attention and action.

Troubled Sex Lives

My clinical work through the years has brought me in contact with many women who were experiencing serious sexual or relationship problems. Sometimes they were aware that their problems had a negative effect on their parenting, but they never mentioned their child's sex education or sexual future. As you read the following case, speculate about the emotions that this woman might feel about her sex life and how such feelings could affect her ability to guide her child on sexual matters.

> Frannie is an attractive thirty-five-year-old woman who came to therapy because her husband Fred wants her to experience orgasm. She says that she is not unhappy with their sex life but might be if she knew what she was missing. She feels her overall relationship with Fred is good, although she doesn't understand why he is so intent on having her experience orgasm.
>
> She explains their lovemaking routine. When Fred pleasures her through manual stimulation and she begins to experience highly arousing sensations, Frannie stops him, thinking that these sensations (and her orgasm) should come through intercourse. Although their subsequent intercourse is pleasurable, she loses her arousal level and does not reach orgasm. Frannie says she knows she is inhibited in that she continues to stop the good sensations, wants the lights off so her husband won't see her body, and worries about making noise during sex because of their thirteen-year-old son in the house.
>
> Regarding their activities as a couple, Frannie mentions that they have never been away alone in a motel, never go out alone for a date, and don't share many

interests. Because they both work and she doesn't like to leave their son home alone, the weekend entertainment is family oriented: going to church, eating out or bringing food home, and watching a video. Frannie and Fred don't see a link between their sexual difficulties and their attitude toward their son's developmental needs, but a couple of questions may provide insight into their situation: What keeps Frannie and Fred from having private sexual opportunities and social activities as a couple? And is Frannie aware of her son's stage of social and sexual development?

You probably discerned that Frannie's inhibitions about sex in her own life are probably spilling over and causing her to deny her son's sexual development and need for sex education. She believed that putting her focus on the family and not on her own sexuality was the best approach. Her discomfort led her to devalue her intimate relationship, give up the idea of private time with her husband, and miss the fact that her son was growing up and not in need of his parents' constant attention.

For some women, the more serious Level II problems with sexuality and intimacy leave them highly stressed and excessively focused on themselves. With their unique sexual identities under attack, they may experience a range of negative emotions: disappointment, embarrassment, disgust, or boredom during sex; shame for having sexual or relationship problems; guilt for not having "normal" sexual functioning; anger toward their partner or themselves; confusion about sexual values and decisions; and despair at finding solutions. Given this ongoing emotional turmoil, they may bypass the task of helping their children with sexual concerns or leave it to hit-or-miss efforts.

Both minor and major sexual problems can drain a woman of energy and enthusiasm for life and render her unwilling or unable to take a rational approach to her child's sexuality. And you have likely considered whether you are currently experiencing any of these sexual concerns or even others not mentioned here. Get ready to go beyond speculation and take the next step toward making an honest evaluation of your sexual relationship.

What You Want and What You Get

People's definitions of a good sexual relationship vary widely. The necessary ingredients can range from a certain level of emotional connection with a partner to a certain level of physical and sensual pleasure. As you would expect, generally several requirements, not just one, make up the wish list. A good way to pinpoint the desired ingredients is to recall a specific, typical sexual experience.

A given sexual encounter exists within a linear time frame, much like that in literary works. The sexual event includes three basic stages: a prologue; the overall interaction itself, which includes a beginning, middle, and end; and an epilogue. The encounter is not, however, simply a linear process. The time frame during which two people engage in sex embodies a great deal of psychological complexity, as both partners simultaneously experience many thoughts, emotions, physical movements and actions, and physiological responses. These reactions, whether or not they are conscious or revealed verbally, influence the moment-to-moment evolution of the couple's sexual experience.

Here's how the sexual interaction unfolds. The prologue sets the tone of the event. Before sex even begins, a lot is happening in the minds of each partner. They both come with a sense of the overall relationship, its tenor and its meaning, all suffused among thoughts and feelings about themselves, their partner, and the bond. The sexual interaction itself encompasses the moment-to-moment unfolding, from beginning to end, of each person's actions and responses, which also include private or shared thoughts and feelings. During the epilogue, after the sex, partners make some sort of mental evaluation of the sexual interaction, which they may or may not reveal to each other. This evaluation becomes one more piece of information that influences each person's sense of the overall quality of the relationship, which they then bring to their next sexual encounter with each other.

At conscious and unconscious levels, people constantly judge the quality of their sexual relationship in a very basic way—namely, they assess what they get compared to what they want. They have in mind expectations for an ideal sexual encounter; then, during the actual interaction and afterward, they measure the reality against the ideal and judge the fit between the two.

The brief Personal Inventory that follows contains the major dimensions of the prologue, the sexual interaction itself, and the epilogue of a given sexual encounter. (At some point your partner should also independently do this exercise, and Chapter Two specifically invites fathers to do so.)

Personal Inventory

Sexual Interaction

Directions. To complete the inventory, recall in as much detail as possible your most recent *typical* sexual encounter with your spouse or committed partner or, if you are not so involved, your most recent *typical* sexual encounter with a partner. Typical means just that: the usual event (not the "once a year" variety at a romantic vacation hideaway). Take time to re-create an image of that experience. Close your eyes and get a picture of yourself, your partner, the time of day, the location, and your verbal and nonverbal exchanges, including what you wanted to say but did not.

As you read each item, ask yourself two questions:(1) What are my ideal expectations for this aspect of the sexual interaction? (2) What actually took place in this recent sexual interaction? Place a plus sign (+) on the line in front of each item if that sexual interaction mostly met your ideal expectations, a minus sign (–) if it did not meet your expectations, and a question mark (?) if you are uncertain. For example, for the first item, suppose that you hope for strong feelings of attraction between you and your mate but did not experience those feelings in the encounter. Your answer would be a minus sign (–). Whereas some items ask for your own internal feelings and thoughts, items pertaining to your partner ask only for your *perception of behaviors* that you could have observed.

Prologue

_____ 1. The attraction, chemistry between my partner and me

_____ 2. Our interest in and affection for each other as persons

_____ 3. Our love, emotional connection, honest sharing of ourselves that bring feelings of being valued and cared for

_____ 4. Our compatibility in life goals, values, interests, dedication to family welfare

_____ 5. Our approach to contraception and (if needed) protection from sexually transmitted infection

_____ 6. Our approach or adaptation to any health or physical limitations that affect our sexual relationship

_____ 7. The typical frequency of our sexual relations

The Sexual Interaction

_____ 8. The timing and environmental setting

_____ 9. The ways and means of initiating sex

_____ 10. My desire, interest, willingness

_____ 11. My partner's desire, interest, willingness

_____ 12. My arousal, excitement, overall sexual responsiveness

_____ 13. My partner's arousal, excitement, overall sexual responsiveness

_____ 14. My level of activity and involvement

_____ 15. My partner's level of activity and involvement

_____ 16. The kind of sexual activities we engage in

_____ 17. My activities to pace and move the sexual interaction toward desired pleasure

_____ 18. My partner's activities to pace and move the sexual interaction toward desired pleasure

_____ 19. My ability to experience intercourse without physical pain

_____ 20. My partner's ability to experience intercourse without physical pain

_____ 21. Our communication during sex

_____ 22. The emotional bond embodied in or communicated during the sexual activity

_____ 23. My orgasmic release

_____ 24. My partner's orgasmic release

_____ 25. Our afterplay, winding down, ending the interaction

Epilogue

_____ 26. My evaluation of my physical, sexual satisfaction

_____ 27. My evaluation of my partner's physical, sexual satisfaction

_____ 28. My evaluation of whether the sex strengthened our emotional bond with each other

_____ 29. My concluding feelings of love, closeness, affection toward my partner

_____ 30. My evaluation of whether the sex strengthened our overall relationship

---

Understanding Your Sexual Relationship

Scoring. Begin by counting (−) responses for items 10, 12, 19, and 23; enter the number on the line for "My sexual functioning." Next, count (−) responses for items 11, 13, 20, and 24; enter the number on the line for "My partner's sexual functioning." Now count and enter the total number of (+) and (−) responses. Finally, determine the ratio of positive to negative responses; for example, if you gave twenty positive responses and ten negative responses, the ratio would be 2:1.

_____ My sexual functioning

_____ My partner's sexual functioning

_____ Total number of (+) responses

_____ Total number of (−) responses

_____ Ratio of positive to negative responses

This brief inventory cannot capture all of the dimensions and nuances of your sexual relationship, but it allows you to render an honest evaluation for yourself, perhaps recording reactions that you have not consciously admitted to yourself or shared with your partner. There are two ways to interpret your scores. First, look at the separate scores on sexual functioning for you and your partner. These pertain to desire, arousal, and orgasm, and to absence of pain during intercourse. Minus ratings on any of these mean that one or several aspects of your own or your partner's typical sexual functioning fall short of your expectations. The presence of a persistent sexual dysfunction for either of you could also have a negative effect on other aspects of the sexual interaction.

Second, compare the total number of pluses to the number of minuses. Obviously, having more minus than plus ratings suggests substantial dissatisfaction with your sexual relationship. A stricter criterion, however, is to see whether your ratio of positive to negative responses is 5:1 or higher. (In the case of this inventory, this would mean that you entered five or fewer negative responses.) This index comes from John Gottman's research, which measured the number of positive and negative interactions within the overall marital (not just sexual) relationships of two thousand couples. Regardless of other factors, satisfied couples were those who maintained the ratio of five positives for every negative interaction in their marriage.[6]

Third, consider whether you had a large number of (?) responses (five or more). Only you know what this response means. It may reflect ambivalence, reluctance to evaluate your sexual interaction, or simply a vague memory of parts of your sexual encounter.

By working through the personal inventories in this chapter, you have taken the pulse of your own sex life. The reasons for doing this are what this book is about: (1) you need to be aware of sexual concerns and problems that produce feelings of unhappiness, dissatisfaction, or ambivalence about your sex life and sexual identity; (2) with awareness, you can overcome these sexual hang-ups and improve your own sex life; and (3) satisfaction with your own sexuality creates a positive, rational attitude and approach toward fostering your child's healthy sexual development. The next section shows how a parent's unhappy love life can interfere with the duty to teach her child about sex and morality.

The Legacy of Inhibitions and Unhappy Sex Lives

Talking about sex in a factual, honest, rational manner remains taboo and unfamiliar to most people. Even for well-adjusted and well-informed adults, a child's sexual question can initially send their emotions into overdrive—surprise, shock, confusion, and embarrassment giving challenge to rational thinking. In the same situation, parents who harbor personal sexual discontent may experience a rush of painful feelings that quickly reaches flood stage.

Helping a child with sexual or moral situations calls for the parent to be knowledgeable, thoughtful, rational, and able to give factual answers suitable for the child's age; to offer a moral perspective; and to lead a sensitive, effective discussion that respects the child's need to know. But what happens when a child's question or situation causes the parent to be deluged by overwhelming negative emotions? A person who is in a highly charged emotional state and experiencing considerable internal psychic pain will not readily think clearly and make good judgments. One common reaction is to escape from the pain by fleeing the scene, avoiding the interaction, or quickly ending it. The parent might respond, "Don't ask such questions" or "We'll talk about that when you're older." But if the parent's emotional state causes her to distort the nature or intention of the child's question, she might respond in more hurtful ways, discharging her unpleasant emotions by directing them toward the child: shaming, criticizing, blaming, warning, or taking a controlling, dramatic stance in giving advice or setting standards.

Besides experiencing unpredictable eruptions of emotionality, the parent with inhibitions or sexual problems may have other qualities that make it difficult for her to approach a child's sex education in a consciously planned and rational manner. Consider the possible legacy from a parent's low self-esteem; dislike of body image or appearance; fear of intimacy; or negative attitudes toward sexuality, one's intimate partner, the opposite sex, people, or life in general. A parent experiencing such burdensome sentiments may lack the willingness, knowledge, confidence, moral authority, and sense of hope and positivism to guide a child toward a healthy sexual future.

The following vignette offers a glimpse of how one mother who struggled with her own sexual problems handled the difficult and complex feelings she experienced as her daughter matured. Keep in mind that her responses were largely unconscious, primarily because she had not faced and consciously resolved her own sexual issues.

As a single mother twice divorced, Allison had felt sexually inadequate and unattractive since her teen years. Although currently dating occasionally, she often felt disappointed with the men she went out with and wondered if she would ever have a meaningful committed relationship. Unconsciously, Allison overidentified with her sixteen-year-old daughter and invested much energy in ensuring that her daughter would be happier in her teens than Allison herself had been. She had given her daughter a few basic facts about sex but was hesitant to talk further, even when her daughter got serious with her first boyfriend. Because Allison herself never got asked out when she was a teenager, she felt happy about her daughter's popularity. In a sense, she was reliving her teen years through her daughter and behaved more like a girl-friend than a mother. Allison became a confidante who uncritically participated in the teenager's near obsession with appearance, weight, clothes, shopping, friends, dates, and boyfriends.

Parents with unresolved personal sexual problems may respond in various unbalanced ways to their child's sexuality. One parent may become permissive and fail to offer needed family rules and supervision. Another may overemphasize the dangers and disap-pointments that sexual and intimate relationships can bring. Still another may become controlling, restrictive, suspicious, accusatory, or excessively protective as the youth matures and seeks greater independence. With their own sexual concerns lurking in the back-ground, such parents often lack the energy to think rationally about what they need to do to guide their child toward a healthy sexual identity.

Parents who have a positive attitude toward sexuality and their own sex life will have the energy to obtain the sexual information that children need and to learn how to talk about it as well. The family factors that seem to influence adolescents to *delay* sexual activity are high-quality parent-child communication about sex (specifically, mutual understanding, listening, and enabling the child to feel understood); a strong, supportive, close, loving relationship between parent and child; and clear communication of sexual val-ues and standards. Thoughtful explanations are especially important in complicated family structures (for example, to prevent children from drawing their own conclusions about parents' dating or intimate relationships).

Such positive family factors don't come easily. They embody communication and relationship skills that call for considerable effort, personal maturity, a high level of rationality, and conscious planning for a child's sex education. Under the best of circumstances, achieving such skills would challenge any parent. How much more difficult it must be for parents who struggle with negative emotions and attitudes due to their own unhappy sex lives! But this conclusion is not the end point. It is the beginning of the next stage of preparation: action and change.

Taking Action: Changes, Solutions, Resolution

Just as our sexuality and sex lives are with us throughout the life cycle, so too is the need to address sexual concerns. Doing what it takes to "make things better" cannot be a one-time event but rather an ongoing part of life, because adaptations are always necessary if we live life fully and long enough. Changes in a person's sexuality are bound to happen as she matures into her thirties, forties, and fifties; and throughout life come changes due to career decisions, health issues, children's maturing, the possible loss of a love relationship and the seeking of a new one. Even slight shifts can affect the self and identity, and these figure into all aspects of intellectual, emotional, and social life, including overall sexual satisfaction. So although the steps I suggest here for finding remedies and resolution might sound like a one-time effort, think of them as a mind-set that will be useful now and in the future.

The key to overcoming hang-ups is basic problem solving. Effective people do this all the time with other dimensions of life—their job, income, living conditions, vacations, children's education, retirement, and so on. They obtain information, read books, consider past and present life goals and personal needs, talk to their partner in thoughtful ways, evaluate options, and use professional advice if needed. Yet, when it comes to their sexual life together (and to some extent their mental health and overall relationship), partners often bypass these steps in solving a problem and simply endure their personal distress.

You, however, are ready to do things differently. Keep in mind the twofold goal: to improve your own sex life and to increase your competence and comfort in guiding your child on sexual matters. Having a positive attitude toward your own sexuality is especially important in talking with young people about the really difficult sexual issues. Otherwise, how can you explain to your teen the ingredients of a meaningful sexual relationship, the right reasons for delaying sexual intercourse, the idea of sexual pleasure for girls, differences in boys' and girls' responses to sex, why both boys and girls need to be "sex-smart," the reasons for noncoital sexual activity, or any other vital sexuality issue?

Now that you have taken inventory of your sex life, it is time to move on to the next step and learn to apply problem-solving skills to your sexual worries, just as you do in other aspects of life.

Level I: Resolving Minor Sexual Concerns

Regardless of the severity of your particular sexual hang-ups, your work on the inventories has no doubt already brought you new insights and increased knowledge that give you a head start on finding good solutions. As you continue reading and interacting with the material in this and other chapters, you can gain important problem-solving and communication skills you can use both to resolve your own problems and to enhance your child's sex education.

The most minor and common Level I sexual problem likely stems from society's and perhaps your family's general taboo about sexuality. This hang-up consists of feelings of embarrassment, confusion, or ignorance with regard to sex. In this case, these emotions are not due to personal dissatisfaction with your sex life or inability to enjoy sex or intimacy with a partner. In other words, you have somehow learned to overcome the taboo and create a good sex life for yourself. What often makes this possible is having an intimate pleasurable sexual relationship, especially with a partner whom you trust enough to reveal your eroticism. Pleasure is a powerful reinforcement for new learning!

Engaging in sex and talking about sex are quite different activities, however. Because adults rarely engage in rational, sustained sexual discussions that bring about a good result (reward or reinforcement for the effort), they don't readily unlearn all the negative emotions that may accompany the process of *talking* about sex. Many adults who enjoy satisfying, pleasurable sexual lives cannot engage in open, honest, focused, and factual sexual talk—whether with partners, other adults, or children. We hope, of course, that this book has already begun to chip away at the emotional barriers that get in the way of talking thoughtfully about sex. But besides increasing your emotional comfort with the topic of sex, there are other action steps to use in resolving Level I sexual concerns.

Before launching into unknown territory, most people like to get a sense of their bearings, specifically their current location, the desired destination, and the surest route. Because succeeding each step of the way is an important principle of learning, the following suggestions begin with those that are likely to be simplest and to cause the least anxiety. You can also choose whatever order and pace seem to best fit your plan for change. For details about specific suggested resources and books, see the section "Adult and Couple Sexuality and Relationship Concerns" in the Resources.

1. *Continue to learn more about the facts of sexuality through a variety of sources.*

- Read an up-to-date book that offers comprehensive coverage of all aspects of human sexuality.

- Read books specifically designed to provide sexual information to children of various ages. (See "Sex Education Resources" in the Resources.)

- View or order informational videos or television documentaries devoted to factual coverage of important sexual issues.

- Obtain sexuality education materials that your school system uses in its sex education programs.

- Obtain sexuality education materials that your religious denomination distributes or uses in its sex education programs.

- Talk with a close friend and your mate about what you are learning about sexuality.

- Read a book that focuses on communication, sexuality, and intimacy in marriage or couple relationships (not simply a book on sexual techniques).

- Read a book on effective parenting and family communication.

- Attend educational or enrichment workshops on parenting, family communication, marriage, problem solving, divorce, stepfamilies, and the like.

- Talk to close friends about this book or form a small discussion group to share sex education materials to use with your children, even if you meet only a few times.

2. *Continue to learn more about your current attitudes and values regarding all aspects of sexuality.*

- Many of the books suggested in "Adult and Couple Sexuality and Relationship Concerns" in the Resources contain sexual attitude inventories for you to complete.

- With any attitude scale that you complete, think about your results and prepare to talk at some future point with your partner, if available, about sexual attitudes.

- Use the discussion of family values in Chapter Three as an opportunity for you and your partner, if available, to take inventory of your sexual values and religious or moral positions on sexual conduct.

- Make a special effort to delve into your attitudes, values, and feelings about sexual pleasure, as these are often a stumbling block in resolving sexual issues.

3. *Review your sexual history.* Approach this review as a personal quest to learn about the many factors that contributed to your sexual upbringing and current sexual identity. Allow several days to a week for this exercise so that you have time to think about your memories. Begin when you have a good block of private time, without interruption, to devote to yourself. Get relaxed and have a notepad handy. In whatever way works for you, recall in as much detail as you can the following aspects of your sexual history:

- Earliest sexual memory

- Earliest information about sex

- Childhood sex play

- How your parents and other family members dealt with sexuality

- What they modeled in terms of affection and intimate relationships

- Sexual messages or information from religion

- Stories of parents' or other family members' dating, sexual behavior, marriages, pregnancies, affairs, divorces, and so on

- Upsetting sexual experiences

- Sexual awareness, experimentation, masturbation

- Factual sex education from parents, school, books, church, friends, partners, media, and other sources

- Misinformation, sexual myths, or sexual stereotypes received

- Crushes, dating behavior, sexual activity with opposite or same-sex partners

- Serious sexual or love relationships, engagement, marriage, committed relationship

- Loss of intimate relationships through breakup, divorce, death

- Personal sexual mistakes, problems, disappointments

This review should bring increased personal understanding and insight that will help you decide if you still struggle with sexual issues from the past. After completing the review, you may want to go further and select certain aspects of your history to discuss with others—your partner, parents, siblings, or a close friend. If you have unresolved family violence or sexual trauma in your history, do not undertake this discussion independently, but work with a qualified therapist first to resolve the trauma and explore the advisability of any disclosures.

Sometimes adults find it helpful to talk with a parent about troubling questions or feelings that they continue to have about their history or sex education. For example, an eighty-year-old acquaintance recently told me that her adult son, at age forty, asked her in a blaming tone why she had never explained wet dreams to him when he was a youth. Their discussion had the effect of improving the overall mother-son emotional bond. She explained that because she grew up in a household of women only, she had no knowledge of nocturnal emissions and had never learned of these even as an adult married woman. Her son gained appreciation of the extent to which sexual taboos controlled his mother and father's generation. Her husband had not shared this information with her or, unfortunately, with his son.

4. *If you are married or in a stable, committed relationship, continue to evaluate the quality of your sexual relationship and determine the steps you wish to take to improve it.* A two-pronged approach is possible with Level I concerns. First, look at your role in the problem and determine changes that you will make independently. Second, look at the parts of the problem that require your partner's involvement in change, and plan to build a joint commitment to improving your sexual relationship. The next two sections discuss these two approaches in more detail.

Level I: Making Independent Changes

Making independent changes is always risky business. Although you believe the changes you make in yourself could bring a good outcome, your partner, unaware of your goal, may react to keep things the same. To succeed, you need to adopt and keep telling yourself the following rational beliefs:

- I am making a change that I believe will help our sex life and overall relationship.

- I am doing something different for myself (not asking my partner to make a change).

- I am taking this action because it's right for me and offers an opportunity for personal growth.

- My effort to change represents a commitment to act on my insight—my truth—whether or not my partner is at the same point.

- I accept that there are no guarantees that my effort will bring the benefit I hope for.

- My idea of success is that I made the effort or took the risk.

These rational thoughts can strengthen you to continue to explore independent change actions. You have already started this process by virtue of interacting with the therapeutic milieu of this book. Armed with new personal insights and commitment to act, you may already have further ideas about changing your steps in the dance of sex with your partner.

Clients often mention that they would like a different tone, time, approach, or type or amount of sexual or sensual activity in their lovemaking with their partner. It never occurs to them, however, to orchestrate the dance more to their own liking, or at least to change their own steps. For example, if you want and enjoy more kissing, you can initiate or sustain kissing. If you want more or a different kind of stimulation or touch, you can guide your partner's caresses. If you find yourself censoring physical, emotional, or behavioral responses that you think would increase your pleasure or your partner's, you can risk showing your true self.

On a verbal rather than a behavioral level, you can also take independent action by sharing with your partner (without asking for participation, cooperation, or a particular reaction) what you have experienced or learned about *yourself* from all the other steps described in the preceding sections—your reading, inventory results, sexual history, and so on. This type of honest, nondemanding sharing gives you practice in talking about sexual issues in a rational manner. It also increases your comfort in doing so and sets a positive tone for future discussions when you seek your partner's cooperation in resolving any remaining or future sexual concerns.

Finally, before jumping into independent changes in the sexual arena, consider whether you might first want to change some aspect of your behavior in your overall relationship with your partner that could strengthen the emotional bond between the two of you. Because general relationship concerns may not elicit as much anxiety as sexual difficulties, these can be a safer starting point for change, whether through your independent efforts or your invitation to engage your partner in joint problem solving. Before delving into your sex life, think about whether any of the following dimensions of your relationship could stand improvement: communication, job and money matters, household routines, parenting duties, leisure, social life, extended family, life goals, or religious or philosophical values.

Level I: Making Changes with Your Partner

Beyond independent efforts, the second approach calls for your partner to work with you to resolve a low-level sexual concern. For example, your results on the "Sexual Interaction" Personal Inventory you took earlier should suggest specific issues in your sexual relationship to bring up. Scores that indicate sexual dysfunctions or pervasive dissatisfaction mean, however, that your relationship may have serious problems (see the next section for resolving this level of sexual difficulties).

Inviting your mate to talk about sexual concerns takes thought, planning, and sensitivity. If you truly want to engage your partner in this joint effort, you need to prepare. Most couples find it difficult to talk about sex, and raising a sexual issue can quickly deteriorate into an exchange filled with personal defensiveness, counterattacks, and withdrawal (recall what happened in Dell and Dan's discussion of their children's sex education). Completing the various action steps described earlier is good preparation for this more complicated step, as is strengthening the overall relationship bond. The following guidelines identify a few rules of effective communication and problem solving to use in talking about a sexual concern with a partner.

- Do not bring up a sexual concern immediately before, during, or after a lovemaking session.

- Explain that you want to talk about some insights or ideas you have about your sexual relationship and invite your partner to have the talk at an agreeable time.

- Explain that your goal is to improve or enrich your sex life, not to have a complaint session.

- Explain that you value your sexual relationship and want the two of you to talk openly about it and see whether you agree about any changes the two of you want to make.

- Start with a specific compliment or affirmation of your partner and the relationship.

- Mention that the two of you may differ in ideas and reactions and that talking about these can strengthen the relationship.

- Give time for your partner to react, and show that you value the response, even if it is negative.

- Express your thoughts in the form of "I" statements that report your own thoughts and feelings. Do not sneak in such "you" statements as, "I think you don't love me." Instead, state your feeling or thought along with pinpointing details; for example, "I feel I could get more turned on to sex if you wouldn't immediately go for my crotch and seem so intent on getting me to orgasm quickly."

- Express your thoughts or concerns in a way that also invites your partner's reaction. For example, follow the concern stated in the preceding point with, "That's my feeling, but what's it like for you?"

- Keep the tone light, even humorous, if that is typical of your style.

- Instead of setting big or specific goals, view your first talk as a way of getting started on a lifetime of more open exchanges about sex.

- Regardless of outcome, stay in a positive mood and show appreciation that you both were able to start talking about your sexual life together.

Here's a sample of how one such conversation went for one couple. Notice how it got off to a bumpy start and then gradually became more comfortable and easy for both partners.

IRIS: Honey, I was wondering if we could talk about our sexual relationship and how it's going.

IAN: You mean now? What's wrong with it?

IRIS: Now is OK unless you want to at some other time. Nothing's wrong. But I think it could be good to talk openly. It could make our love even stronger and the relationship better.

IAN: I sure don't have any complaints.

IRIS: Me neither. It's not about complaints. Sometimes I'd like to share more with you, but I just hold back. So I decided to go out on a limb and be more open. You might even like what I have to say—or even get turned on.

IAN: Getting turned on is not a problem for me. Is it for you?

IRIS: It's not usually. But I have some thoughts about how our sex might be better for me—and I wonder if you ever have ideas that you think about but never say.

IAN: You surprise me. You go first.

IRIS: Well, sometimes I feel like it would be exciting for me to get things started and seduce you, but I feel like I never get the chance. Seems like you want sex more often than I do, so I end up just reacting to you.

IAN: Maybe I'm just hornier than you.

IRIS: Maybe, but we'll never know for sure this way.

IAN: I guess I do just think it's my job to get things started. Maybe I worry that if I don't, we won't.

IRIS: I get turned on once we start, and I enjoy what we do. You're a great lover. You do make me feel good—in lots of ways.

IAN: I guess I knew that, but it's nice to hear you say it.

IRIS: There is one other thing.

IAN: Uh-oh. Now the bombshell!

IRIS: No way. Sometimes though, I think we're in too much of a hurry. It feels like we're getting into a routine. Like sometimes, I want to be on top with intercourse. I think I would get different sensations that way. I feel funny just saying that out loud to you.

IAN: That's fine. I think I'd enjoy it if you were more active. In fact, can I say something? You won't get mad?

IRIS: What have I done here, created a monster? Go ahead. I guess it's my turn to listen.

IAN: Sometimes I feel that you avoid my penis, except for when we start intercourse. That's just my feeling, maybe because you don't touch it or you just do it quickly and go on to something else.

IRIS: Well, I never thought about that. I guess I don't touch it, and I guess I don't even look at it either. Maybe I'm not so liberated after all. But I do like it when you press it against me.

IAN: Like I said, I think our sex is fine. But I'd like you to touch me more—say, in more teasing ways.

IRIS: This is interesting. I've learned something about myself here, and you too.

IAN: Are you OK with what I said? I hope so.

IRIS: It's fine. You're my lover boy. We should be able to say anything to each other.

IAN: Where do we go from here?

IRIS: Who knows? But not to the bedroom! I'll deal with you later.

This interaction shows how one woman invited her partner to talk about their sexual relationship. After recovering from some initial tension, this couple got off to a good start. Such talks don't have to be lengthy or end with specific goals or proposed changes. By ending on a positive note, as Iris and Ian did, you will be encouraged to be more open, which will make it easier to generate more ideas and changes to try. Your future talks and efforts to do things differently may even become more spontaneous. And remember to tell each other when you notice any improvements.

It's a giant stride to be able to talk together to resolve a sexual concern. Remember, moving in this direction not only helps you get the sex life you want but also strengthens you to help your child achieve a healthy and happy sexual future.

Level II: Resolving Serious or Complicated Sexual Problems

Serious or complicated sexual hang-ups can lead parents to neglect their children's sex education or lace it with negative or confusing messages. Recall the Personal Inventory "Level II Sexual Concerns," which listed the more serious individual sexual and relationship problems. There you indicated whether you experience any of these problems and whether you need to resolve them.

Individual or couple counseling from a mental health professional is advisable for any of the serious problems that you may have checked for yourself. You should also seek professional help for any of the lesser concerns that don't improve through your own individual or couple efforts.

If you recognize that your intimate or sexual life is in disrepair, unraveling, or even ripped apart, you can benefit from professional therapy, regardless of the decisions or outcomes that may result. Taking the step to enter therapy requires commitment—both to improving your own sex life and to fostering your child's future sexual health. If you keep these two end goals in mind, you can enter the process and work at it, even though there is no guaranteed outcome.

Therapy for Problems in Marriage or a Committed Relationship

The dynamics that create and maintain complex problems in a couple's intimate and sexual relationship often have multiple roots. These include each partner's family of origin, personality, attachment needs, negative thinking, disturbed moods, and self-defeating behaviors. On their own, people are rarely able to change the rigid interaction patterns that bring so much unhappiness.

Couples with children in middle and high school often struggle with meeting their own individual and relationship needs along with the increasing demands of these childhood stages. In attempting to juggle so many needs, parents may ignore their own intimate relationship. This pseudosolution produces unresolved discontent that can affect how they approach their child's need for sexual and moral guidance.

What happens is that just when your child most needs your rational and thoughtful guidance, your unhappy love life may leave you feeling unloved, unappreciated, and depleted of energy. Dealing with your child's emerging sexual maturation is stressful under the best of conditions, but consider how burdensome this parental duty might feel if you are not coping with the rest of life's demands. For example, here are just a few of the common pressures that go with this stage of life:

- Demands and setbacks related to job, career goals, and finances

- Demands from children's expanding school, social, and community activities

- Stress associated with moving to a new home or locale

- Needs of aging parents and in-laws

- Health problems of your own, your partner, or your child

- Ambivalence or concerns about aging

Under too many of these conditions, partners may not nurture their sexual and love relationship, perhaps assuming that it will survive to see a better day. In fact, some couples can make this turnaround happen. Unfortunately, others make no changes, and the relationship may continue, stable but unhappy. Often because the partners don't believe in or wish to divorce, they settle into a state of malaise and disenchantment with their marriage. Such a choice takes a toll, however, on both family life and each partner's mental health.

Therapy can help uncover a common dynamic at the heart of some of these troubled marriages, specifically, partners' unconscious, irrational expectations. For example, we often enter a marriage assuming that a partner will fulfill our fantasy of the ideal mate, meet all of our needs, heal wounds from our family of origin, boost our flagging self-esteem, or manage all of the family's crises. We can learn that marriage cannot do for us what we must do for ourselves: discover and cultivate our own sense of value, competence, attractiveness, and worth as a whole person.

With professional help, partners can often gain a more logical vision of their relationship and see options other than enduring unhappiness and resentment. Depending on their unique situation, several outcomes can represent a good resolution of problems. Partners may agree to try out new behaviors or communication skills to strengthen their relationship, see some good results, and end up renewing their bond. Change of this sort, however, is not the only way to improve a relationship and one's mental health. In some situations, partners find a good resolution when they come to understand and accept that certain of their individual qualities, in themselves or in their partner, may not change or may not need to change. Another option that some couples choose—usually as a last resort—is to end an unhealthy intimate relationship that is unresponsive to their sincere efforts to make improvements.

Therapy for the Concerns of Single Mothers

Some of the problems that affect single mothers can be especially distressing. Even if mothers are happy or optimistic about their dating life, intimate sexual relationship, or cohabiting relationship, complications can arise with regard to a child's feelings and attitudes about these aspects of Mom's life. Women in these situations (particularly if all is not well with their sex life) need a high level of awareness. They need to maintain appropriate boundaries between their own life and needs and their child's. They should strive for a sense of congruence between their personal values and behaviors— what is right for their own sex life. They should decide what standards of sexual conduct they want to pass on to their child and talk about these openly. Depending on their own dating and intimate relationship and whether these are apparent to the child, they may need to explain further if and why the child's standards do not apply to Mom as an adult. It is much better to think about these issues in advance rather than have your child say, "How can you tell me that sex belongs in marriage when you don't live by that rule?"

The dynamics involved in a single mother's sexual identity and approach to intimate relationships can be complicated. Therapy is useful in identifying the many sources involved in self-defeating patterns and emotional turmoil.

A major issue pertains to a mother's own needs for an intimate relationship. Many important questions go unanswered for many women in this circumstance:

- Have I resolved the effects of losing my previous love partner and learned from the experience?

- Have I recovered from any damage to my self-esteem due to this loss or other losses?

- Do I have a healthy approach to my needs for a social life and companionship?

- What are my motives for and expectations of dating relationships?

- What are my values with regard to sex in dating relationships?

- What are my values with regard to cohabiting with a partner?

In addition to their own personal lives, single mothers have to cope with other family responsibilities such as job, finances, and parenting (possibly coparenting with an ex-spouse). A common question that arises is how to meet their own personal needs while also being aware of and meeting their children's developmental needs. Therapy can help women sort out this issue and find answers that fit their child's age, personality, and current adjustment. Without an objective viewer to prod for rational analysis, certain blind spots can persist. A recent client, while in the process of a long, drawn-out divorce, became angry when her husband took their four-year-old son to play with the children of his current affair partner. Yet several months later and with no progress toward the divorce, she and a male companion began to include her son on their picnics and other outings. She simply couldn't see the similarities between her own behavior and that of her husband.

There are no pat answers for how single parents, both mothers and fathers, should handle and explain their dating or intimate relationships so as to meet their children's best interests. Children's sexual and emotional development becomes increasingly complex during early puberty and adolescence. To make wise decisions, parents need to think about and reach answers for several questions, some of which they may not yet have acknowledged:

- How do I explain to my child my interest in exploring new relationships?

- How should I present and conduct my dating activities?

- Should my child meet my dating partners?

- Should my sexual activities take place in my home?

- Should my child participate in "quasi-family" activities with my dating partners?

- What if my child becomes attached to dating partners who then disappear?

- How should I present my serious love or committed relationship to my child?

- How should I explain adult dating or intimate relationships compared to adolescent relationships?

- What sexual standards and expectations do I wish to set for my child?

- How can I account for or resolve any incongruence between my own adult sexual standards and those I expect of my child? Can I find the words to explain this to my child, if an explanation is needed?

- If I have a live-in relationship or remarry, how should I deal with family rules for privacy, maintaining personal sexual boundaries, possible feelings of attraction to new family members, and other such issues?

Obtaining Professional Help

Therapy can be essential to help parents explore these and other questions. For the more serious problems, professional help can promote both personal awareness and workable solutions. The first, most practical issue is finding the right kind of professional who is competent to work with your problem. Careful thought and inquiry should definitely go into this decision, and the following guidelines may help.

1. Consider whether medical factors may figure into your sexual problems and whether to start with a physical or gynecological examination.

2. Ask your physician's opinion about the type of professional you should consult, such as sex therapist, couple therapist, psychologist, psychiatrist, social worker, mental health counselor, or pastoral counselor.

3. Call or write professional associations that certify specialists in such areas as marital and family therapy and sex counseling and therapy. (See "Organizations and Internet Information Sources" in the Resources for detailed listings and contact information for the major certifying associations.) Other good sources for referral information are local universities (especially those with medical schools), mental health professional training programs, and good reference libraries.

4. Ask for a referral from a trusted professional in your community or from friends who have been in therapy.

5. Obtain firsthand information from several recommended professionals before setting an appointment. Prepare a list of questions to ask in a phone conversation or letter—about the person's professional degrees, specialized training and credentials, experience with sexual concerns such as yours, approach to treatment and therapy, fees, and the like. A competent and qualified professional will gladly respond to these and other questions.

A final question may be whether to take some independent steps before or even during therapy, such as those listed in the sections on dealing with Level I concerns (reading about sexuality, exploring one's sexual history, making independent changes, talking to one's partner). Only you can make this decision. Knowing the severity of your problems, you can decide whether you have the energy or optimism to carry out some of these action steps. If you go forward on your own and achieve benefits, you can take that as a sign that you should continue independent efforts.

————————

From this chapter you have learned how to identify your own sexual hang-ups and take action to find remedies. Your happier sexual life will leave you with more positive emotions about your own and your child's sexuality. As your feelings of shame, confusion, inadequacy, fear, and vulnerability decrease, you will no longer sense the strong impulse to avoid your child's sexuality or respond with emotional reactions such as avoidance, lectures, warnings, condemnations, and so on. You can then approach this aspect of parenting with the calmness, rational thinking, and planning that you give to your other parenting duties.

Further groundwork lies ahead. Chapter Two enables fathers to take inventory and take charge of their own sexual hang-ups. Chapter Three talks extensively about how you and your partner (if both of you are available) can join as teammates in guiding your child toward sexual health.

2

Taking a Personal Inventory for Dads

*We are now in a period of crisis. Every man who is
acutely alive is acutely wrestling with his own soul.
The people that can bring forth the new passion, the
new idea, this people will endure. Those others, that
fix themselves in the old idea, will perish with the new
life strangled unborn within them. Men must speak
out to one another.*

D. H. Lawrence, Foreword, Women in Love

While writing this book, I talked about it with a friend, the
father of two young boys. This young man told me that he
hoped to teach his kids about sex, recalling that he hadn't received
any information or guidance from his own dad or mom and didn't
really know where to begin, but would gladly read this book or
attend a group educational program for parents to learn how to do
it. I believe that many other fathers share this sentiment, but perhaps don't quite know what to do.

This chapter is a good starting point, and it specifically addresses
dads (although moms are welcome to listen in). Even if you're not a
dad or you have sent your young adults out into the world, you know
other men who are fathers. Maybe you have talked with them about
kids growing up and the worries that come with that. This book will
put you in a good position to help your own son or daughter with

sexual matters. But you should also consider sharing your insights with other fathers you know who are having a hard time with this.

The idea of doing things differently can be daunting; we often wonder if we have the know-how to try something new. A good way to start any new process is by taking inventory of what we already know and what we need to learn. To become involved in your child's sex education, the first step is taking inventory of your own sex life. This includes more than your sexual relationship with your wife or significant other. Even if you are not in an ongoing intimate relationship, you still have a sex life to review. After doing this, you can decide whether your current sex life suits you and meets your needs or whether you would like to make some changes. The bottom line is that learning more about your own sexuality is the first step to becoming your child's sex educator and moral guide.

Dads' Avoidance of Their Child's Sex Education

Both fathers and mothers have critical roles to play in their child's sex education and moral development, but dads have often stayed on the sidelines. Some men, no doubt, do have meaningful talks with their children about sex. And when these take place, kids value and benefit from the ideas and advice. Nevertheless, many fathers, just like mothers, have unconscious sexual hang-ups that make them very anxious about the prospect of talking to their kids about sex.

The anxiety strikes in unexpected situations. One dad was shocked to hear his ten-year-old son use the word "testicles." The boy had been to the doctor for a skin rash, and when his older brother asked where the rash was, he simply replied with the correct terminology. His dad told him he should say "privates."

Perhaps you have had similar experiences. Maybe, for example, the idea of talking openly about sexual facts just doesn't seem right.

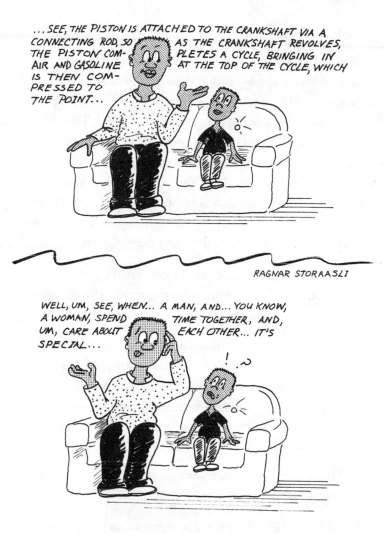

Or you find yourself avoiding your son's sexual questions. Or you worry about your daughter's sexual life and decisions but do nothing. Get ready to change that old pattern. This chapter empowers you to review your own sex life and your thoughts about your child's sex education. Once you uncover the source of troubling feelings and thoughts, you can use your insights to overcome sexual hang-ups.

Men's Experience with Sex Education

The sexual hang-ups of men differ from those of women. For start-ers, men often accept as normal their minimal role in their child's sex education. This myth seems to persist even for dads who take an active part in all other aspects of parenting. The reasons are understandable. When these men were themselves young boys, they were unlikely to have experienced their own dads giving them good information about sex; having had no model, they gained no sense of this being part of their job as fathers. The questions that follow will help you recall your sex education: how much you learned and whether you saw respected and trusted men carrying out this role.

- Did you get accurate, factual information about sex in school, church, or community programs? (Were there any male teachers or leaders?)

- Did you learn, from any authoritative source, about the range of human sexuality (sexual organs, physiology, behaviors, reproduction, contraception, pregnancy and childbirth, STDs, intimate relationships, differences in responses of boys and girls, sexual orientation, pornog-raphy, sexual offending, and so on)?

- Which parent, if either, gave you factual information about sex?

- Did he or she talk to you about sexual morality and standards of behavior?

- Did you feel understood, supported, and respected by your father? By your mother?

- Were your father and mother appropriately affectionate with you?

- Did you go to your father or to your mother (or neither) for advice about sexual and relationship matters?

- Did you agree with your father's sexual attitudes and values? With your mother's sexual values?

- Did you feel that your father and mother would have stood by you if you had had a serious problem with sex?

- Did you have any serious sexual problems as a teenager or young adult?

- Who or what was your most important source of good information about sex?

- Who or what were the sources of misinformation or attitudes about sexuality that were not helpful or added to your worries about sex?

Understanding Your Inertia

By thinking about your answers to these questions, you can learn why you might "shut down" in regard to your child's sex education—why you can't get past the uncomfortable feelings, why you may lack confidence, why you may be all too willing to let Mom do the job. I believe that the most common sexual hang-up among dads is a bad case of inertia.

The reasons for this stance are not mysterious. First and foremost, people learn behavior from imitating other people's behaviors that bring an obvious reward, such as a good outcome, expression of thanks, or positive human interaction. If you didn't have the experience of seeing your own father or other adult men talk to kids about sex, you may not automatically jump in and do this for your child. At the same time, you may take a look at the world children are growing up in today and decide that you want to guide them on sexual matters. Doing this job may not come naturally, but your good intentions can be turned into action to learn how to do it.

There are some barriers to overcome. As we've discussed, a lot of men (and women) have simply never seen fathers in the role of talking to their kids about sex. Consequently, much of society continues to maintain the status quo: "fathers need not apply." In fact, mothers who have had uncomfortable or hurtful sexual discussions with their own fathers may consciously exclude their child's father from sexual situations that arise in family life. They may wish to protect their child from a similar experience, or they may assume they can do the job better than the father in the household.

A second reason for fathers' "bailing out" has to do with another principle of learning: avoidance breeds more avoidance. Here's how it works. When painful emotions arise in a given situation or in thinking about that situation (such as feeling ignorant about a child's sexual question), getting rid of the pain becomes paramount. The readiest response is simply to avoid the situation or thinking about it. In so doing, what we learn is to keep avoiding the same situation. The sad thing is that as long as we keep reacting in this way, we also avoid the opportunities that make new learning possible.

Fathers' Emotional Maelstrom

Men's sex lives and history are at the heart of the intense feelings that strike when they face the prospect of their sons' and daughters' sexuality. This topic somehow seems at odds with paternal sentiments of love and protection. When there are so many dangers and so few real solutions, a father can begin to feel overwhelmed.

At the root of this confusion are feelings that may never quite become conscious. In fact, because of their social programming, many men don't pay much attention to their inner emotional life. They become so adept at repressing feelings that they are not aware of *experiencing* them. Yet they pay a toll for this kind of short-lived relief. For example, in the vignette here, a father's "gut-level" feelings seem to be dictating his approach to his son's sex education.

> At age forty-five, Alex had experienced a couple of episodes of erectile dysfunction. Instead of talking with his wife, trying to recall whether he might have had too

much alcohol on these occasions, or asking a physician about the problem, he began to avoid sexual relations with his wife, blame her for the problem, and fantasize that all would be well with another woman. Sometimes when he looked at his seventeen-year-old son, he felt both sadness and envy. He saw his own sexual life as taking a downhill track while his son was bursting with sexual energy and attractiveness. Alex gave no thought to offering his son sexual information. His own parents had never talked to him about sex. He figured that boys find out what they need to know, and in his heart he almost hoped that his son would "get as much sex as he could."

With effort, you can change patterns that lead to avoidance of your child's sex education. By completing the inventories in this chapter, you can gain understanding of your feelings about sexuality, your own sex life, and your child's sex education. Further suggestions offer ways to cope with difficult emotions, turn negative thoughts into more rational ones, and change aspects of your life if you need to. When these burdens lift, you can expect greater self-acceptance, increased personal comfort with sexual topics, and a new willingness to improve your knowledge of sexuality. No longer will you need to shun meaningful discussions about sex with your partner or child.

Men and Stereotypes of Male Sexuality

The normative socialization of most men throughout childhood and youth produces attitudes and behaviors that affect their sexual life. As is true for women, our culture has some pretty rigid ideas of how men should approach their sexuality. We tend to learn these ideas automatically, simply because they surround us, not by choice. Before further exploring male gender roles, see if the following two-part inventory sheds light on your sexual life or helps you better understand men in general.

Personal Inventory

Sexual Pleasure and Male Roles, Part I

Directions. Answer the questions keeping in mind your marital relationship or, if you aren't married, your current committed relationship or, if you aren't in a committed relationship, your most recent ongoing sexual relationship. Place your answer in column A. Later you will come back and add an answer in column B.

                                                                    A   B

1. How many times during a typical, average day do you have a pleasurable sexual thought, fantasy, image, or genital sensation?   _____   _____

2. How many times during the course of a typical month do you experience sexual desire or interest on your own (not in response to your partner's desire)?   _____   _____

3. How many times during the course of that typical month do you act on your own desire by initiating sexual activity with your partner, in a very direct way, verbally or physically?   _____   _____

4. How often do you typically experience orgasm when you engage in sexual activity with your partner? (Rate on the following scale: 0 = 0 percent, 1 = 25 percent, 2 = 50 percent, 3 = 75 percent, 4 = 100 percent of the time when engaging in sex.)   _____   _____

5. Would you like to experience orgasm more often? (0 = no, 1 = yes)   _____   _____

6. Have you ever clearly told or shown your partner the kinds of touch, caress, activity, or stimulation that you enjoy or that bring you the most pleasure or to orgasm? (0 = no, 1 = yes)   _____   _____

7. How many times in the past six months did you masturbate and reach orgasm alone?   _____   _____

A   B

8. Rate the physical and sensual gratification you derive
   from sexual activity in a typical sexual encounter with
   your partner. (0 = none, 1 = a little, 2 = some, 3 = a lot,
   4 = completely satisfied)   _____   _____

9. Rate the psychological and emotional satisfaction
   you derive from sexual activity in a typical sexual
   encounter with your partner. (0 = none, 1 = a little,
   2 = some, 3 = a lot, 4 = completely satisfied)   _____   _____

Now go back to each item and in column B rate the amount of anxiety
or embarrassment and discomfort that you experienced in answering each
item. Use the following scale: 0 = none, 1 = a little, 2 = some, 3 = quite a bit,
4 = a great deal.

Scoring. Add all the numbers on the lines in column A to arrive
at your total item score. Next, add all the numbers in column B,
which rates your anxiety, to arrive at your anxiety score. You can
enter these scores here:

_____ Total item score

_____ Anxiety/embarrassment/discomfort score

Interpreting your Part I scores. Part I of the inventory is highly
focused on only a few aspects of your sexuality. It is not an indicator of your overall satisfaction with your sexual or intimate relationship. So, that said, what can it tell you?

The *total item score* reflects your level of sexual desire, the degree
to which you are motivated to act on it, and the value you place on
physical and sensual sexual pleasure. Are you satisfied with your
level of desire? If so, are you satisfied with your frequency of acting
on it? If not, is it something about you or the relationship or your
lifestyle that keeps you from initiating sexual activity? Are you satisfied with the level of physical pleasure that you receive from your

sexual encounters? The lowest possible score is 0, which suggests a total disinterest or disavowal of sexual desire and pleasure. Another negative scoring pattern consists of high numbers on sexual desire and interest (questions 1, 2, and 5) but low numbers for acting on or achieving sexual pleasure (questions 3, 4, 6, 7, and 8). On these five items, the higher numbers mean that you take greater initiative to experience sexual pleasure and that you derive physical satisfaction from your sexual activity.

The *anxiety score* reflects the amount of negative emotion that you feel about your level of sexual desire and the physical pleasures of sex. Is your anxiety high for the questions about independent sexual desire? Is your anxiety high for the questions about the pursuit of pleasure (masturbation, orgasm, physical gratification)? A total score between 0 and 10 suggests very little negative emotion; 11 to 20 suggests some; 21 to 30 suggests quite a bit; and 31 to 40 suggests a great deal of negative emotion. The idea here is to *reflect* on what these numbers mean for you. Do they cause you to think about your sexuality in a different way? Do they enable you to face some personal concerns that you typically ignore or avoid?

Personal Inventory

Sexual Pleasure and Male Roles, Part II

Directions. Consider the following beliefs about men and their sexuality. In column A, rate the extent to which you accept the belief, using the following scale: 0 = not at all, 1 = somewhat, 2 = quite a bit, 3 = completely. In column B, indicate how often your behavior in your sex life tends to mirror these beliefs. Use this scale: 0 = never, 1 = occasionally, 2 = often, 3 = always.

	A	B
1. Men are pretty much always interested in sex.	___	___
2. Men readily get into the pleasures of sex without holding back.	___	___

	A	B

3. Men get easily aroused and ready for sex.   _____ _____

4. Men are the experts when it comes to sexual
   know-how.   _____ _____

5. A good erection is essential for good sex.   _____ _____

6. Men are expected to initiate sex with a partner.   _____ _____

7. Men are mostly in charge of directing the activities
   and positions during sex.   _____ _____

8. Men are responsible for their partner's sexual
   satisfaction.   _____ _____

9. Men's main focus during sex is on intercourse
   and orgasm.   _____ _____

10. Men are expected to perform as sex partners.   _____ _____

Scoring. Add all the numbers on the lines in column A to arrive at your total belief score. Next, add all the numbers in column B, which reflects how often your behaviors tend to mirror the beliefs, to arrive at your total behavior-beliefs score. You can enter these scores here:

_____ Total belief score

_____ Total behavior-beliefs score

Interpreting your Part II scores. For column A, a score from 0 to 10 means that you are not a strong believer in these ideas about male sexuality; a score from 11 to 20 means just the opposite, that you tend to accept them. For column B similarly, a score from 0 to 10 means that your behavior in your sex life does *not* tend to mirror these beliefs; a score of 11 to 20 suggests that your behavior in your sex life *does* tend to mirror these beliefs.

As you look at your scores, think about what the numbers mean for you. Do they remind you of sexual concerns that you usually don't think about or attempt to resolve? The next section looks further into the stereotypes about male sexuality and what gives them power.

Men and Nonrelational Sex

In general, society pretty much accepts that sexual desire and sexual satisfaction are "normal" for males. But the whole experience of growing up male can leave men strongly predisposed not only toward sexual fulfillment but also toward *nonrelational* sex. Obviously, not all men get the exact same dose of social programming, so they, like women, will vary in their approach to love and intimate relationships.

Nonrelational sex is based on lust that is unconnected to a real or imagined partner who has value as an equal subject. Instead, without any fixed requirement for a relationship or emotional intimacy, the person values the partner simply as a sexual object or vehicle to orgasmic satisfaction. Psychologists Ronald Levant and Gary Brooks argue that men's disposition toward nonrelational sex is manifested in what they call the "centerfold syndrome," which is a "pervasive distortion in the way men are taught to think about women and sexuality."[1] The resulting attitudes and behaviors can damage men's inner emotional life, relationships with women, and sense of masculine worth.

> Ben was a client who was caught up in this belief system at an extreme level. At age forty, he had been involved in a series of three or four affairs following recovery from a heart attack. After meeting women in bars, he would quickly get into sexual relationships. He expected his wife to accept his current affair, as he had no plans to end it. Ben admitted in therapy that he was looking for a good time, not for an emotional relationship. Throughout his decade of marriage, material success had been his obsession. His wife was his business partner, and she felt

that their marriage was nothing more than a perfunctory partnership. Unresponsive to his wife's needs for affection and intimacy before and during this period, he also remained oblivious to any of his own emotions or needs that might be triggering his affairs, such as feelings of vulnerability and fear of death resulting from his life-threatening illness.

Men and Traditional Masculine Roles

Nonrelational sex is an extreme result of men's social conditioning; other attitudes are much more common and likely to affect a dad's involvement in his child's sex education.

> Although totally opposite from Ben in most ways, Carl still had a hang-up when it came to his kids' sex education. He was a devoted and faithful husband, and he and his wife Cathy both greatly enjoyed their sexual relationship. But when Cathy began to ask him to help her with sexual information and rules of the house for their fifteen-year-old daughter and twelve-year-old son, Carl told her that she should do it, because she had already talked with their daughter several years ago. But he was quick to remind Cathy not to be so easy on the kids, not to get bogged down in listening to everyone's feelings, and to simply lay down the law. Cathy wondered to herself how Carl could be so uninhibited sexually with her and still feel so uncomfortable at the thought of talking with the kids about sex. She had hoped he would at least do some of this for their son, but that didn't happen.

The attitudes and values that push some men toward nonrelational sex can also affect men who never behave this way. Early on, boys get a lot of cultural messages that shape their personality and identity in many ways. Specifically, self-styled "gender police" (peers, coaches, parents, teachers, the media) enforce the so-called boy code to get boys to comply with the traditional masculine gender role.[2] Consequently, to varying degrees, boys learn to

- Suppress and give no voice to the softer emotions

- Repress needs for care and connection, especially from their mother

- Channel complex emotions into the response of anger

- Lose touch with their inner life

- Avoid talking about their feelings and problems

- Value self-reliance and personal control

- Pursue achievement and status

- Objectify and devalue girls

- Pursue sexual gratification to fill the vacuum created by the loss of meaningful connections to others

Carl had apparently absorbed much of this kind of learning, and it had followed him right into adulthood and marriage. Living out his traditional upbringing, he accepted that sex is very private, that it is not to be talked about and is certainly not a subject that kids need to know much about. Carl also believed that listening to kids' feelings and worries is not a good approach to parenting and may be a form of spoiling kids when parents need to be in charge. Other factors may be linked to his reticence; for example, he may feel some shame about his own teenage sexual behavior or lack of knowledge about the details of sexuality.

Boys who end up following "the code" lead a very limited emotional life. As teens and young men, they may begin to measure their worth in terms of conforming to these notions of masculinity. They automatically learn to look to their peers for how well they are doing as "real men." What brings respect and reward are such behaviors as toughness, being in control, fixating on women's appearance and body parts, boasting of sexual conquests, denigrating homosexuals, and avoiding any personal qualities or activities that smack of "femininity." Adolescent boys with strong needs to fit in often engage in these behaviors even when their true self rejects them.

Research results support this hypothesized social construction of men's sexuality. For example, a recent large-scale study of sex in the United States found that compared to women, men hold more permissive sexual attitudes, engage in more recreational sex, have more sexual partners, and engage in more varied sexual experiences. Similarly, other findings have reported that men differ from women in masturbating more frequently, buying more autoerotic materials, and having more explicitly sexual fantasies.[3] Obviously, not all men are cast from this hypermasculine mold that says "more sex is better," but it affects all of us in some ways—both men and women.

Male Stereotypes and Becoming a Father

Understanding male socialization is a starting point for appreciating the psychological dynamics behind men's avoidance of their child's sex education. I am most concerned for men who get wide exposure to these rigid attitudes without ever seeing them challenged. What do they experience when they become fathers? They will probably have strong sentiments of joy and hope when their offspring arrive, and respond with feelings of love, nurturance, and protection. When a child is young, they may never even think to compare their day-to-day fathering with their own sexual history or sex life. That changes, however, when a child approaches puberty and dads consciously recognize (if only for a brief moment) that their son or daughter will have a sexual life. At this point, they often begin to draw parallels (if only for a brief moment) between their own sexual life and the sexual future that awaits their child.

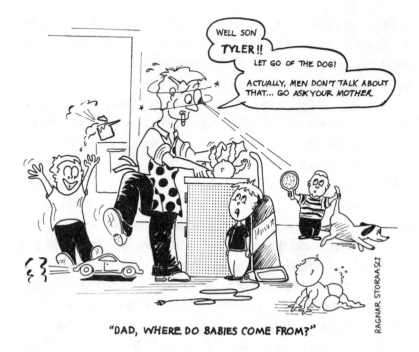

"DAD, WHERE DO BABIES COME FROM?"

This momentary insight can bring a surge of confusing emotions that erode optimism about their child's sexual future, perhaps especially so for their daughters. Folk wisdom puts it this way: the reason fathers want to lock away their teenage daughters is that they know from experience what teenage boys are like.

Whether or not a father experiences this kind of reaction will likely depend on the degree to which he lets rigid masculine stereotypes dominate his thinking. If he is happy with both his sexual life and his moral life, he should be able to see both the positives and negatives of his child's coming of age. Better still, if he begins to talk with others, such as his child's mother, he can overcome his reluctance and be a part of his child's sex education.

Tracking Deeper-Level Feelings and Thoughts

At this point, you have an opportunity to explore a variety of possible emotions and thoughts that may trigger your avoidance of your child's sex education. Some negative feelings and thoughts may arise even if you personally enjoy a satisfying sex life and consciously reject stereotyped notions of masculinity.

Personal Inventory

Men's Thoughts and Emotions Elicited by Their Child's Need for Sex Education

Directions. Imagine yourself needing to talk with your child about a sexual matter or being asked by your partner to do so. Imagine this situation with your child both younger and in adolescence. If you have more than one child in these age groups, select the child whose sex education worries you the most. Briefly close your eyes to get a vivid image of that situation. Then, as you read each emotion and each thought in the inventory that follows, decide whether you experience any of these emotions or thoughts (or similar ones) as you imagine the situation. In front of each emotion and corresponding thought, place the rating sign that best fits what you experience when imagining these situations. Use the following scale: plus sign (+) = applies to me a lot; minus sign (–) = does not apply to me at all; question mark (?) = uncertain.

Emotions	*Thoughts*

Early and Middle Childhood

_____ Embarrassed	_____ I don't know enough. I'll mess up or it won't go well.
_____ Anxious	_____ Sex is too personal and private. I don't want to get into that.
_____ Annoyed	_____ My kid is too young. It's not necessary now.

Puberty and Adolescence

_____ Sad	_____ My kid is growing up, but I'm getting old. We'll lose the fun and innocence of childhood. The teenage years will be hard.
_____ Overwhelmed	_____ There's too much to cover. I can't say everything in this talk.

Emotions	_Thoughts_
_____ Embarrassed	_____ I don't know enough or how to talk about sex and feelings and right and wrong. I'll look stupid. My kid will be uncomfortable. Kids think they know everything about sex anyway.
_____ Awkward	_____ My kid will be uncomfortable getting into this personal stuff (and so will I).
_____ Irritated	_____ Kids get this stuff in school; they can figure it out for themselves; they think they know it all anyway. Mom can handle this.
_____ Worried	_____ It's a scary world—drugs, AIDS, rape, violence, gangs. It was easier when I grew up. I can't protect him [her].
_____ Sad	_____ My kid will probably have hurt and disappointment too. I can't be of much help.
_____ Ashamed	_____ My own sex life is not that good, and I don't know how to fix it.
_____ Confused	_____ I can't even fix or run my own sex life. I'd be a hypocrite trying to explain sex and tell my kid how to behave.
_____ Ashamed	_____ I've made my share of sexual mistakes. I'm not a model for success or virtue. I don't want to think about this.
_____ Guilty	_____ I've got my own sexual skeletons in the closet. (I've objectified, used, hurt, exploited, coerced, or raped partners; done some "weird" sexual stuff; risked the welfare of myself, partners, a committed relationship, marriage, the family through some of my sexual behaviors.)
_____ Humiliated	_____ I'm not that great as a sexual partner. I don't have a good sex life even now. Kids hear all

Emotions	Thoughts
	about Viagra and make jokes about it. They know adults don't have much of a sex life going.
_____ Fearful	_____ What if my kid asks about my sex life? I've got to keep this under wraps. I might let something slip out.
_____ Hopeless	_____ My sex life will never be any better. I haven't got anything to offer my kid. Nothing ever turns out right anyway.

Scoring. Count the number of pluses, minuses, and question marks for the Emotions column and then for the Thoughts column. You can enter them here:

Emotion Totals	Thought Totals
(+) _____	(+) _____
(–) _____	(–) _____
(?) _____	(?) _____

Interpreting your scores. Because all these emotions and thoughts are negative, a higher number of pluses means more negative reactions; a higher number of minuses means fewer negative reactions; a high number of question marks means you are not sure whether these emotions and thoughts describe you. Note also that the last seven emotions and thoughts in the inventory reflect negative feelings and thoughts linked to personal sexual hang-ups.

This exercise offers only a few speculations about men's emotions and thoughts. The idea is to help you explore what goes on in your mind and heart. Were you able to identify, at least to yourself, whether hang-ups about the topic of sex in general or your sexual history might relate to uncomfortable emotions and negative thoughts about your child's sex education? Certainly, your reactions will depend on how well you have resolved your own sexual issues and whether you were thinking about a son or a daughter or both.

Men's Sex Lives

Several research findings support the speculations about men that appear in the inventory you just took. For example, recent studies show that boys today report more gaps in their sexual knowledge than girls. They also believe that girls know more about sexuality than they do. Teenage boys further report that they get into relationships before they are ready to manage them. In addition, they often acknowledge that their first experience of sexual intercourse was a disaster because of their ignorance.[4]

Considering that these findings describe boys in the 1990s, the current generation of fathers would have had even less exposure to factual sexual information. These fathers also likely got a strong dose of social programming toward hypermasculinity and overvaluing of sexual performance and conquest. With these characteristics, today's fathers probably experienced their share of past sexual disappointments as well. Some of them may also face current sexual difficulties.

Recent research from a large-scale study of sex in the United States has suggested that 31 percent of men experience sexual dysfunction. This total represents such problems as lack of interest in sex, inability to achieve orgasm, premature ejaculation, erectile disorder, lack of pleasure, and anxiety about performance. Two problems increase with increasing age: trouble achieving or maintaining an erection (18 percent at age fifty to fifty-nine) and low sexual desire (17 percent at age fifty to fifty-nine). Problems showing similar percentages within four age groups (eighteen to fifty-nine) include inability to achieve orgasm (range of 7 to 9 percent), early ejaculation (range of 28 to 31 percent), sex not pleasurable (range of 6 to 10 percent), and anxiety about performance (range of 14 to 19 percent).

Considering that only about 10 percent of men with such problems seek medical consultation, we must conclude that many men simply endure these kinds of complaints.[5] Media accounts about new drug treatments, such as Viagra, have brought the topic of male sexual dysfunction squarely into public view. Although positive in some ways, this attention has also given way to a spate of jokes (especially on the Internet), thus adding to feelings of inadequacy for men who experience sexual difficulties.

Conforming to stereotypes of masculinity, such as hiding weaknesses or personal problems, can compound men's sexual difficulties and prevent them from finding rational solutions. Many men opt for the status quo rather than take steps to learn the full facts about sexuality or their particular sexual problem. (Remember the point that only 10 percent of men sought professional help for a sexual complaint.) At the same time, they are likely to put more pressure on themselves by overvaluing sexual performance and believing that they must be an expert in seducing and satisfying a woman.

As you learned in Chapter One, some of mothers' personal sexual concerns can elicit highly charged emotional reactions when they contemplate their child's sexuality. The same is true for fathers. This is why you need to continue taking inventory of your sex life.

In this last evaluation exercise, the focus was on your feelings and thoughts in the context of your child's sex education. This approach addressed what I stated is the most common hang-up of fathers: inertia. That is, they so accept the idea of being a marginal figure in their child's sex education that they rarely even think that scary emotions are behind their avoidance. By this time, you have become aware of the feelings and thoughts that the topic of sex education brings. And at this point you are ready to take a deeper look at the very personal worries that relate to your sexuality, behaviors, and intimate relationships.

To determine whether any sexual difficulties are keeping you from having a happier sex life, you will need to complete several inventories. The first covers the more common sexual worries that most people have from time to time.

Personal Inventory

Level I Sexual Concerns

Directions. Put an X in front of any item that is a concern you currently experience and a second X on the line if you need to resolve the difficulty. For example, you might need to resolve a problem if it causes negative emotions, thoughts, or behaviors that interfere with your sense of well-being or the kind of intimate and family relationships that you want. Resolving such a difficulty could entail changing behaviors or adopting more rational or balanced thoughts and attitudes, such as letting go of past mistakes or forgiving yourself. Conversely, some of the problems that you experience many not be sufficiently relevant or distressing to affect your life situation or choices.

_____ 1. Lack of sex education or sexual knowledge that leaves me feeling ignorant or inadequate

_____ 2. Shyness or timidity in communicating with my partner or child about sexual matters

_____ 3. Past sexual choices and behaviors that I regret or feel guilty about

_____ 4. Dissatisfaction with aspects of my body, features, or overall appearance

_____ 5. Ambivalence about my sexual values

_____ 6. Lack of congruence between my professed sexual values and actual behavior

_____ 7. Uncertainty, as a single father, about how to handle my dating and intimate relationships in regard to my child

_____ 8. Confusion about the sexual values and moral code I want for my child

_____ 9. Current sexual choices and behaviors that I regret or feel guilty about

_____ 10. Unwanted or excessive sexual inhibitions within my committed relationship

_____ 11. Unresolved shift in my personal sexual values, beliefs, or conduct (for example, from liberal to conservative or vice versa)

_____ 12. Occasional questions about my sexual orientation

_____ 13. Unresolved feelings about women in general as unfairly receiving advantages because of their gender

_____ 14. Discomfort, embarrassment with the sensual or physical aspects of sexual pleasure

_____ 15. Discomfort, annoyance with the emotional, romantic aspects of intimate relationships

At this point, a quick count of the double X's can suggest whether one or more difficulties are keeping you from having a happier sex life. (Later you will return to these when you're ready to take action to resolve them.) You can further evaluate the quality of your sex life by considering the more distressing sexual and relationship problems. People often put up with an unhappy love relationship, sexual dysfunction, or unwanted sexual behaviors and, consequently, simply suffer in silence. These kinds of problems take a toll on a man's overall sense of happiness and well-being. Acknowledging and facing up to such problems is the first step toward achieving real solutions. To learn more about yourself, consider whether any of the disturbances in the following list trouble you.

Personal Inventory

Level II Sexual Concerns

Directions. Put an X in front of any problem that you currently experience and another X if you need to resolve the problem. For example, you might need to resolve a problem if it causes negative emotions, thoughts, or behaviors that interfere with your sense of well-being or the kind of intimate and family relationships that you want. Resolving such a difficulty could entail changing behaviors or adopting more rational or balanced thoughts and attitudes, such as letting go of past mistakes or forgiving yourself. Conversely, some of the problems that you experience many not be sufficiently relevant or distressing to affect your life situation or choices.

_____ 1. Sexual dysfunction (problem with desire, arousal, or reaching orgasm in the way or time frame desired, or pain during sex) in myself or my partner

_____ 2. Severe overall dissatisfaction in my marriage or committed relationship

_____ 3. Cheating by me or my partner in a relationship based on fidelity

_____ 4. Unresolved childhood or adult sexual trauma for self or partner

_____ 5. Incongruence and dissatisfaction with the sexual orientation or gender identity that I or my partner present to the public

_____ 6. Sexual disorders in myself or partner, such as unwanted sexual fetishes or criminal sexual offending

_____ 7. Problems in adjusting to the loss of my partner through divorce, death, disability, or ending of the relationship

_____ 8. Inability to find or maintain acceptable dating partners or the kind of intimate relationship that I want

_____ 9. Sense of despair or disgust toward all sexual and intimate relationships

_____ 10. Indiscriminate, risky, or compulsive sexual behavior.

A count of the double X's can suggest whether one or more of these serious difficulties are keeping you from having a happier sex life. (Later you will return to these when you're ready to take action to resolve them.) Having completed the last two inventories, you will likely have a sense of whether you harbor some minor or major sexual hang-ups that deserve your further attention and action.

Level II problems not only bring stress for your own life but also can drain away your energy and good intentions to help your child with sexual concerns. The same is true if you harbor a lot of dissatisfaction in your current sexual relationship—whether with your spouse, committed mate, or other occasional or regular sexual partner.

What You Want and What You Get

People have different ideas about what makes a good sexual relationship, and men and women may or may not differ in this. Sometimes the issue centers on how much emotional exchange and how much physical and sensual pleasure feel right. Although you may not have given this subject much conscious thought, a good way to evaluate your satisfaction is to recall a specific, typical sexual experience.

A sexual encounter has a time frame: a beginning point, the interaction itself, and an end phase. But a lot more than the passage of time takes place. While both partners are engaging in actions and movements, they are simultaneously experiencing their own thoughts, emotions, and physiological responses, which they may or may not share with each other.

Here's how the sexual interaction unfolds. At the beginning point, before any sex, partners come with their thoughts and feelings about the overall relationship, its tenor and its meaning, along with feelings about themselves, their partner, and the bond. During the sexual interaction itself, more thoughts, feelings, sensations, movements, and physiological reactions happen all at once, as the partners sense each other's moment-to-moment sexual experience or actually share that (or some of it) verbally with each other. After the sex, some sort of evaluation usually takes place, whether or not the partners reveal it to each other. Once this sexual event is over, partners may bring these final thoughts, to some degree, into their next sexual encounter with each other.

At conscious and unconscious levels, people constantly judge the quality of their sexual relationship in a very basic way—namely, they assess what they get compared to what they want. They have in mind expectations for an ideal sexual encounter; then, during the actual interaction and afterwards, they measure the reality against the ideal and judge the fit between the two.

The brief Personal Inventory that follows contains the major dimensions of the prologue, the sexual interaction itself, and the end phase for a given sexual encounter. (At some point your partner should also independently do this exercise, and Chapter One specifically invites mothers to do so.)

☞ Personal Inventory

Sexual Interaction

Directions. To complete the inventory, recall in as much detail as possible your most recent *typical* sexual encounter with your spouse or committed partner or, if not so involved, your most recent *typical* sexual encounter with a partner. Typical means just that: the usual event (not the "once a year" variety during a vacation or trip away from the kids). Take time to re-create an image of that experience. Close your eyes and get a picture of yourself, your partner, the time of day, location, and your verbal and nonverbal exchanges, including what you wanted to say but did not.

As you read each item, ask yourself two questions: (1) What are my ideal expectations for this aspect of the sexual interaction? (2) What actually took place in this recent sexual interaction? Place a plus sign (+) on the line in front of each item if that sexual interaction mostly met your ideal expectations, a minus sign (–) if it did not meet your expectations, and a question mark (?) if you are uncertain. For example, for the first item, suppose that you hope for strong feelings of attraction between you and your mate but did not experience those feelings in the encounter. Your answer would be a minus sign (–). Whereas some items ask for your own internal feelings and thoughts, items pertaining to your partner ask only for your *perception of behaviors* that you could have observed.

Prologue

_____ 1. The attraction, chemistry between my partner and me

_____ 2. Our interest in and affection for each other as persons

_____ 3. Our love, emotional connection, honest sharing of ourselves that bring feelings of being valued and cared for

_____ 4. Our compatibility in life goals, values, interests, dedication to family welfare

_____ 5. Our approach to contraception and (if needed) protection from sexually transmitted infection

_____ 6. Our approach or adaptation to any health or physical limitations that affect our sexual relationship

_____ 7. The typical frequency of our sexual relations

The Sexual Interaction

_____ 8. The timing and environmental setting

_____ 9. The ways and means of initiating sex

_____ 10. My desire, interest, willingness

_____ 11. My partner's desire, interest, willingness

_____ 12. My arousal, excitement, overall sexual responsiveness

_____ 13. My partner's arousal, excitement, overall sexual responsiveness

_____ 14. My level of activity and involvement

_____ 15. My partner's level of activity and involvement

_____ 16. The kind of sexual activities we engage in

_____ 17. My activities to pace and move the sexual interaction toward desired pleasure

_____ 18. My partner's activities to pace and move the sexual interaction toward desired pleasure

_____ 19. My ability to experience intercourse without physical pain

_____ 20. My partner's ability to experience intercourse without physical pain

_____ 21. Our communication during sex

_____ 22. The emotional bond embodied in or communicated during the sexual activity

_____ 23. My orgasmic release

_____ 24. My partner's orgasmic release

_____ 25. Our afterplay, winding down, ending the interaction

Epilogue

_____ 26. My evaluation of my physical, sexual satisfaction

_____ 27. My evaluation of my partner's physical, sexual satisfaction

_____ 28. My evaluation of whether the sex strengthened our emotional bond with each other

_____ 29. My concluding feelings of love, closeness, affection toward my partner

_____ 30. My evaluation of whether the sex strengthened our overall relationship

---

Understanding Your Sexual Relationship

Scoring. Begin by counting (–) responses for items 10, 12, 19, and 23; enter the number on the line for "My sexual functioning." Next, count (–) responses for items 11, 13, 20, and 24; enter the number on the line for "My partner's sexual functioning." Now count and enter the total number of (+) and (–) responses. Finally, determine the ratio of positive to negative responses; for example, if you gave twenty positive responses and ten negative responses, the ratio would be 2:1.

_____ My sexual functioning

_____ My partner's sexual functioning

_____ Total number of (+) responses

_____ Total number of (−) responses

_____ Ratio of positive to negative responses

This brief inventory cannot capture all aspects of your sexual relationship, but it lets you record your reactions in an honest, conscious way. There are two ways to interpret your scores. First, the separate scores on sexual functioning for you and your partner pertain to desire, arousal, and orgasm, and absence of pain during intercourse. Minus ratings on any of these mean that one or several aspects of your own or your partner's typical sexual functioning fall short of your expectations. The presence of a persistent sexual dysfunction for either of you could also have a negative effect on other aspects of the sexual interaction.

Second, compare the total number of pluses to the number of minuses. Obviously, having more minus than plus ratings suggests substantial dissatisfaction with your sexual relationship. A stricter criterion, however, is to see whether your ratio of positive to negative responses is 5:1 or higher. (In the case of this inventory, this would mean that you entered five or fewer negative responses.) This index comes from John Gottman's research, which measured the number of positive and negative interactions within the overall marital (not just sexual) relationships of two thousand couples. Regardless of other factors, satisfied couples were those who maintained the ratio of five positives for every negative interaction in their marriage.[6]

Third, consider whether you had a large number of (?) responses (five or more). Only you know what this response means. It may reflect ambivalence, reluctance to evaluate your sexual interaction, or simply a vague memory of parts of your sexual encounter.

———————

The personal inventories in this chapter have enabled you to take the pulse of your own sex life. The reasons for doing this are what this book is about: (1) you need to be aware of concerns about sexuality in general and personal sex problems that produce feelings of unhappiness, dissatisfaction, or ambivalence; (2) with awareness, you can overcome these sexual hang-ups and improve your own sex life; and (3) satisfaction with your own sexuality creates a positive, rational attitude and approach toward fostering your child's healthy sexual development. The next section shows why these points are so important: they can get you on the right track to begin your important role in your child's sex education.

Dads on the Front Lines

As a father who is preparing to take an active role in his child's sex education, you may have questions about doing this job: Will I be mostly involved with my son? How can I be helpful to my daughter on sexual matters? What do kids need to know and when? This book answers all those questions and more. But at this point let's consider the unique contribution that dads can make.

Fathers need to know that they are important in their child's sex education. They may not totally believe this, as they probably haven't seen models for this behavior and so haven't seen its benefits. My own recent study of adolescent sexual behavior provides encouraging information.[7] A subsample of ninety-nine young adults (ages eighteen to twenty-one) who had not engaged in sexual intercourse during adolescence (defined as ages eleven to seventeen) reported on their reasons for the decision, on their communication with their fathers, and on other aspects of family life. We found that youth who had higher levels of communication with their father (often talking "about almost anything") were more likely to give realistic reasons for avoiding intercourse (expressing concerns about pregnancy, STDs, reputation, and maintaining respect from their partner) and to cite values (personal, parental, religious, and relationship standards) as reasons for avoiding intercourse.

In addition, those who cited values as a reason for remaining a virgin were more likely to have parents who voiced and lived by high moral standards and who were active in church attendance and activities. These findings suggest that teens' reasoning and decisions may benefit from communication with fathers specifically and from seeing both parents' moral and religious commitment in action.

As a father, you also have an influence on all aspects of your child's development, personality, and behavior. This influence will play an important role in whether your child acquires certain characteristics that are associated with healthier sexual decisions. Long before getting into detailed sexual discussions, you can foster the following qualities that promote sexual health in your child: having and pursuing academic goals and achievement; believing in future life goals; participating in religious or community life (or both); having friends who share healthy sexual and moral values; maintaining contact with positive adult role models; holding a clear set of values and moral standards; and following guidelines for good mental and physical health, especially avoiding such risks as alcohol, tobacco, poor diet, and lack of exercise.

Boys are typically shortchanged when it comes to sex education. But because fathers know about men's sexuality firsthand, it seems natural that they should pass on this information to their sons. From the inventories you worked on at the beginning of this chapter, you should know whether you have negative feelings and thoughts about the whole process of your child's sex education—in other words, some hang-up that makes this task one you want to skip. Now you have a chance to get more insight into possible sexual issues that make you most anxious. The following inventory, which focuses on typical sexual concerns of boys, enables you to take stock of your comfort level, knowledge level, and willingness to talk about these topics.

Personal Inventory

Sex Education Topics for Boys

Directions. Imagine yourself about to or needing to talk with your son about the following topics—not just one big talk but many brief talks and comments—starting with the stage of puberty (about age ten or eleven) and through the teen years as needed. Consider each topic and rate yourself on your current comfort level, knowledge level, and willingness to talk about the issue.

Use the following rating scale. Assign a number from 0 to 5 that best describes you at this point in time: 0 = very low, little, poor—very inadequate for this topic; 5 = very high, positive—very adequate for this topic

Topic	My Comfort Level	My Knowledge Level	My Willingness Level
1. The penis—naming, hygiene, size	_____	_____	_____
2. Erections, wanted and unwanted	_____	_____	_____
3. Nocturnal emissions (wet dreams)	_____	_____	_____
4. Masturbation	_____	_____	_____
5. Physical development, appearance, size	_____	_____	_____
6. Sexual harassment (name-calling, objectifying, violating personal space, jokes) of any person, female, male, straight, or gay	_____	_____	_____
7. Sexual molesting (touching, grabbing a person's sexual parts or areas)	_____	_____	_____
8. Sex-related violence against others (coercion, control, hitting, rape—of strangers, dating or steady partners, and persons because of sexual orientation)	_____	_____	_____
9. Being assertive in protecting self and others from sexual harassment, molesting, violence	_____	_____	_____
10. Nature and meanings of sexual intercourse	_____	_____	_____

Topic	My Comfort Level	My Knowledge Level	My Willingness Level
11. Different meanings of sexual intercourse for boys and girls	____	____	____
12. Abstinence as protection against pregnancy and STDs	____	____	____
13. Other forms of protection against pregnancy and STDs	____	____	____
14. Sexual fantasies	____	____	____
15. Pornography	____	____	____
16. Boys' intense emotions (lust, attraction, love, loss, anger, aggression)	____	____	____
17. Questions about sexual orientation	____	____	____
18. Personal morality and responsibility in sexual situations	____	____	____
Total Scores	____	____	____

Scoring. Add the numbers in each column to get your total comfort, knowledge, and willingness levels for dealing with these typical concerns of boys. A total score of 45 on any of these levels suggests overall a middle or average ability. Scores below 45 suggest lower levels; scores above 45 suggest higher levels of ability. Pay particular attention to topics on which you rated yourself below a 3 on either comfort, knowledge, or willingness. These scores indicate a need for improvement.

Fathers should put effort into simply "beefing up" their knowledge about sexuality in general. From reading and talking with a partner about the information, you can quickly gain confidence. There's no substitute for knowing the facts and having a command of the right "language." Think about how you handle other tasks where your reputation is on the line. For example, most men don't go into a work setting to give a presentation or make a "pitch" without good preparation. With the task of sex education, your child's life and future are on the line.

The more you learn about sexuality, the more you will realize that assisting your son need not come solely from discussions, although these are important. Having in mind a single big "sex talk" that must impart everything a kid needs to know would drive any parent into a panic. Giving up this notion and learning how to draw on resources, you can make sure that your son gets all the sexual information and guidance that he needs, when he needs it. (Chapter Three shows parents how to work together as a team for this purpose, including using all the resources that the community offers as well; it also helps you clarify your moral beliefs and values about sexuality so that you will be clearer on the message about morality that you want to convey to your child.)

At this point, I want to discuss the unique contribution that you can make to specific aspects of your child's sexual development—first for sons and then for daughters. (My including certain topics and ideas here does not imply that they are exclusively the responsibility of fathers.) This discussion will enable you to continue taking inventory of yourself and your reactions to the proposed activities, such as father-son and father-daughter talks.

What Fathers Can Tell Their Boys

As you probably guessed from the inventory you just completed, there are certain aspects of sexuality that have been missing in the sex education of most boys. What's more, many of these topics are not in school sex education programs. Because of this, boys need at least one good sex education book that addresses young people. But fathers should also talk about these sensitive issues that worry boys.

You can offer a positive and personal understanding of male sexuality and correct misinformation and distortions that your son may have heard. The discussion that follows doesn't convey every aspect of sexuality that a boy needs to know, but it does suggest how you can be more open in conveying both knowledge and healthy attitudes about some sensitive issues. As you read, ask yourself whether you got this information as a youth; if not, why not; and how your teen years and after might have been different with this knowledge.

The Penis and Secondary Sexual Characteristics

You can reassure your son about several basic facts with regard to the penis and later pubertal development. The suggestions here are not comprehensive and focus on only a few aspects of male sexuality (among many) that often lead to distortions and negative emotions. You can help prevent these. The first tasks listed are the simpler ones and should begin when the child is quite young:

- Teach the correct names for the genitalia. (This does not mean ridiculing other terms your son might have heard or used.)

- Explain how to wash and keep the genital areas clean to protect health.

- Give assurances at all ages that his sexual organs are adequate and will continue to develop. Elaborate, as your son gets older, to dispel myths about penis size and men's and women's sexual satisfaction.

- Acknowledge that touching the genitals is pleasurable but is a private activity.

- Explain that he has the right to decide whether a sexual touch is appropriate and who is allowed to touch his sexual organs. Teach him the skills for protecting himself from inappropriate touch and not to allow violations of his or another person's sexual boundaries.

- Be positive, supportive, and complimentary about your son's growth, development, physical appearance, and personal qualities. Don't tease or allow other family members to tease.

Nocturnal Emissions

Once your son has the basic facts (either from books or parents) about his sexual organs and how sperm and semen are formed, you can explain that nocturnal emissions (wet dreams) are one way the body releases semen during sleep. Nocturnal emissions may or may not be connected to a sexual dream. If your son remembers a dream, he should know that all dreams are normal, regardless of their content.

Reassure him that wet dreams happen to all boys and men, that the semen is not urine, and that he should not worry about this or be ashamed of it. You can also tell him that clothes or sheets are readily washed with the rest of the family laundry.

Erections

Fathers are in a good position to explain the adolescent boy's reality of the ever-present, ever-pressuring erection. Tell your son that this normal physiological response does not necessarily signal the desire for sex or sexual release. A boy needs to know that this response comes and goes, just as does the perennial morning erection (without necessarily calling for any action on his part) and that these unpredictable, automatic, and often unwanted erections will subside as he gets a bit older.

This information introduces the idea that your son is in charge of his sexual response and that desire and arousal do not dictate automatic action to achieve orgasm. He needs to know that he makes a choice to have sexual release, but the decision to start and stop, even in midstream, is his. No dire consequences result if he decides not to act on an erection.

Boys should hear that erections also come with feelings of excitement and arousal. These responses are part of growing up, as is the desire to experience sexual pleasure through masturbation. Let him know that feelings of arousal may be particularly strong during adolescence; there is nothing wrong with masturbating; it has no bad effects; it should be done in private; and he is entitled to privacy. Reassure him that masturbating or not masturbating has nothing to do with a person's masculinity, sexual orientation, ability to attract a partner, or emotional maturity. (Masturbation is also common during adult life.)

Finally, explain that these are the facts about masturbation that should make it a pleasurable experience and leave him feeling OK about himself. In general, masturbation is not a great solution for dealing with loneliness, sadness, or low self-esteem. The result might be greater isolation, which prevents finding real solutions, such as making friends, talking with others about problems, and engaging in enjoyable, rewarding activities that boost self-esteem.

Reproduction and Contraception

From a young age, a boy needs to know that his penis is part of his reproductive system, not simply a vehicle for pleasure. Birth control and pregnancy are among the topics that boys report as gaps in their sex education. Before puberty, they need to understand that managing their potential to cause pregnancy will be their responsibility throughout life. Clearly tell your son that young people should never risk pregnancy, as that creates a life crisis for everyone involved. Let him know that his current goals are to achieve maturity, education, and job skills that will help him realize his life goals, and that causing a pregnancy places his whole future life, as well as that of his partner, at risk.

Concrete and dramatic examples are best for bringing home this point—again and again. A sex education program for boys titled Wise Guys has boys guess the number of grains of sand in a thirty-two-ounce jar (two hundred million to four hundred million), which corresponds to the number of sperm in the typical ejaculation. They also learn that it takes only one sperm to fertilize the female egg.[8]

Use these kinds of down-to-earth examples to help your son begin to realize that with these odds for pregnancy, he should never "blow off" the facts and his responsibility. Myths and stereotypes abound about pregnancy, contraception, boys' part in preventing unwanted pregnancy, the impact of pregnancy on their lives, and impregnation as a sign of masculinity or virility. For example, boys hear such false notions as that girls can't get pregnant during their period, if they stand up during or after intercourse, if they douche with Coca-Cola, and so on. You clearly have your work cut out for you in this area.

Talk about the ways of preventing pregnancy and sexually transmitted diseases. Although Chapter Three will help you consider the moral and ethical position you want to convey to your child, here you can think about the facts of abstinence, birth control methods for women, birth control methods for men, and about the ability of young people to take responsibility for themselves and their partner. Abstinence is effective as long as a person carries it out. Sometimes, however, young people who endorse this value engage in other sexual activities that lead them to unintentionally abandon abstinence; as a result of being uninformed and unprepared, they often have unprotected intercourse. (As a parent you will need to decide on your moral position on abstinence and talk openly with your son about it.)

If young persons cannot imagine themselves talking in detail to a partner about protection, who will get it, how they will use it, what they will do if it fails, and what their intercourse means, they are not ready for sexual intercourse. All of this talk is necessary, and a boy should never assume that protection is up to the girl. He is responsible for protecting both himself and his partner, whether she wants that or not. Tell him that if a girl says that protection doesn't matter, he should stop sexual activity and beware. (As a parent, you will need to decide on your moral position regarding the use of birth control and condoms and clearly let your son know where you stand.)

Differences in the Meaning of Sex for Boys and Girls

Recent research on how boys and girls and young adults approach sexual intercourse shows differences that have long been part of our cultural makeup. Boys often believe that girls should set the limits on sexual activity and that intercourse is acceptable without strong affection, emotional involvement, or commitment. Girls tend to value these qualities more than boys and often agree to sexual intercourse because they want to show their love, please their partner, or strengthen a relationship. When partners have different ideas about why they would have intercourse and what it means, there's room for trouble and disappointment or worse. Young men need to hear from their fathers about these differences and the importance of honesty and communication if a couple decides to engage in any sexual activity. Without this, partners may hold quite different expectations of each other and what the relationship will be like after intercourse.

Aside from discussing the physical risks of intercourse, help your son understand the emotional risks as well. Intercourse carries many meanings, and these may vary for boys and girls. For a boy it may represent a new stage in his sexuality, a new experience in the adventure of growing up. He may associate it with pride and maturity, or even status among peers. Help your son recognize that intercourse is an intimate act involving two people and that this is what makes it both special and complicated. It takes maturity and resources to handle this kind of intimacy with its many risks to physical, emotional, and psychological development. Here is what one courageous father told his eleven-year-old son:

It's not just girls who can get hurt in sex. You have to be old enough and mature enough to know what to expect of yourself and of a girl. To a boy, having intercourse might mean the same thing as masturbating, in other words, a high point loaded with excitement and pleasure. A girl may think it means you love her, want to go steady, want to get engaged, want to marry her. It takes time to learn all of these things. Until you're able to sort out all of these complicated puzzles about relationships that baffle even adults, masturbation is a way to experience that pleasure privately—until you're ready for the "big show" that lasts your whole adult life.

This certainly is a good beginning, and it accomplishes several goals. If this father hadn't broached this subject when his son was this age, he couldn't begin to say this to him when his son was sixteen. This father's words include facts, standards, rules, respect, and a positive attitude toward sexuality. His talking to his son also models that men can talk seriously about sex. Finally, it sets the stage for more discussions to come.

One additional point about intercourse: teach your son the meaning behind some of the peer pressure to engage in intercourse. He is likely to hear that getting a girl to have sex is a status symbol, a sign of manhood. Another myth is that a "real man" should be able to obtain sexual gratification through intercourse under any circumstances, regardless of age, physical or emotional maturity, understanding of his own body, understanding of sexual relationships, interest in intercourse, having a meaningful relationship with the partner, or even having consent of the partner. Help your son reject such myths and conduct his life according to his own values and what is best for him in his life. He doesn't have to wear the straitjacket of stereotyped masculinity that can create doubt and shame about his sexuality and worth.

Sexual Fantasies

Sexual fantasies, daydreams, images, and memories often seem to have a life of their own. These are normal as they come and go, moving freely in and out of our minds; they are also normal when we consciously call them up. They can be highly sexual, romantic, on the "wild side," or all of these. Let your son know that fantasies are just that and are not the same as behavior. At times most people will have a fantasy that they don't like, such as those that include persons, acts, or situations that might seem strange or weird. Fantasies can be a problem if a person becomes obsessed with a particular one or acts out a dangerous or degrading fantasy.

A more complicated issue is that of fantasy with masturbation. Fathers have personal experience that can provide insight into this very private dimension of sexual life. You certainly don't need to be intrusive, but offering some opinions is legitimate. You might simply offer a monologue on people in general (preferably while transporting your son somewhere so he cannot escape), in an informational tone that would not call for a response from him. You could explain that men often masturbate in response to a daydream or fantasy about sex, nudity, or a desirable person and that this is normal.

Young people are surrounded by images of attractive males and females throughout the media. No one has to go in search of these. So it is understandable that images of actors, models, entertainers, and celebrities—the so-called beautiful people—could readily enter a person's fantasy. Fathers can let their sons know that these images are part of our culture and may be part of fantasies, but they are just that—fantasy. Tell him that a media image is not a real, whole person with a life and an identity. Tell him that real people don't look like celebrities, but they have value because they are real people. Tell him that a real lover, partner, or spouse will have exciting qualities and appeal that encompass much more than physical appearance.

Pornography

Pornography is readily available in our culture, especially in magazines, on the Internet, in so-called adult videos and adult sex stores, and other venues. The "adults only" label is often meaningless, as every child today and in the past has likely seen such materials. Fathers (and mothers) need to learn more about the ever-expanding pornography industry that produces materials that go way beyond what they may have seen in their youth. Today's pornography can expose kids to the routine degradation of women and men, all manner of violence linked to sex, children used as sex objects, and worse.

Explain why and what you object to in pornography; put this in terms of the ethics or moral values you believe in. Your son needs to hear this from you. Then explain why the family has restrictions on television, movies, video games, the Internet, and other media. Explain why you expect him to stay away from so-called hard-core pornography. Aside from your moral position, looking at the issue in terms of the psychological development of youth, you can mention that exposure to certain kinds of sexual images (dehumanizing, bizarre, degrading, violent) can shape a young person's total sexual identity without his even being aware of it. These images can rob him of his own individuality. A boy can develop and discover his unique character only by having had time to get answers for highly personal questions:

- Who am I? What are my abilities, talents, and goals?

- What are my inner desires and needs?

- What qualities do I find attractive in a possible partner?

- Who is a real (not fantasized) person who attracts or excites me?

A boy benefits from time to work on these questions, before his psyche and spirit have become entrenched in extreme fantasies (reinforced by masturbation), such as images that dramatically depart from the norms of real life, people, and relationships. If he learns to experience his sexuality in the context of images that objectify and degrade people, depict sexual offenses, glorify bizarre sexual acts, or link sex to violence, his sexual psyche may be on a destructive track. Such unconscious conditioning can be especially powerful when it is part of masturbation. It could affect his sexuality in a variety of unhealthy ways. For example, becoming fixated on such fantasies may make it difficult for him to have satisfying sexual intimacy with a real partner.

Managing Intense Emotions

Public events of the past few years have begun to explode the "macho" myth that only girls battle overwhelming feelings that can send them spinning out of control. Recent school shootings and murders reflect the tragedy of adolescent boys who vented their intense emotional pain, not with words, but through self-defeating and horrendous violent acts.

In their heart of hearts, fathers know about the powerful emotions that can overtake a body and soul. These include unexplainable feelings of lust or "horniness" directed toward people who are unsuitable or unattainable. Or a youth may feel intensely attracted to someone for obvious and not so obvious reasons, such as an older person, stranger, teacher, coach, friend's girlfriend, male friend, and so on. Boys need to know that such emotional reactions are part of growing up and figuring out their own sexual identity and the kind of person who attracts them. They should understand that much of their emotional life is and should be in a state of flux. This is reason to hold off on dramatic or impulsive actions and decisions. Everyone remembers the first (and second or third) crush that one year later triggers puzzlement, shame, or laughter. You can talk to your son about both enjoying such feelings and managing them so as to avoid unnecessary hurt. The same applies to feelings of inadequacy and rejection in relation to achievement or peers. Boys need their parents to help them learn that these reactions come and go throughout life and to help them find healthy ways to cope with them.

Parents who talk with and spend time with their son would know if he has qualities that increase his risk for depression or aggression. If so, they can then provide support or professional counseling to help him cope with losses and disappointments that come with adolescence.

Feelings of attachment and love are complex for boys, just as they are for girls. Fathers (and mothers) can help, but talking about these experiences calls for great sensitivity and support. Contrary to the myth, adolescent boys can and do experience strong feelings of "romantic" love and emotional connection toward a partner. Teenage partners sometimes form sincere relationships that involve their total developing identities. Dating and time spent together serve to intensify their feelings. The couple may be best friends, share interests and goals, and show support and care for each other. Still, such relationships, as all adults know, are fragile.

Once a relationship of this caliber is under way, you can show empathy and approval for your son's caring and regard for his partner. Ideally, information and advice would have come earlier, to let a boy know what to expect—what most people experience:

- Young people may "fall in love" and feel deep affection for a partner; such feelings are to be treasured.

- Boys and girls and men and women often have several such relationships before they are ready to have sex or make a lifetime commitment.

- The end of a relationship brings hurt and pain. People learn that this loss does not mean personal rejection or loss of worth. They learn to manage the pain and continue with life, and it helps to talk to friends or family. Bittersweet experiences are part of the adventure of life, including in adulthood.

Sexual matters are but a few of the more sensitive issues that you can help your son understand. In the best of circumstances, your conversations will not start with a blank slate, as your son would know some facts about sexuality and relationships through school sex education classes, books, or earlier talks with you and his mother. With this foundation, you can concentrate on having follow-up talks that convey such important messages as these:

- Both benefits and responsibilities come with sex and growing up.

- You have reason to be proud and optimistic about your sexual development and future.

- You will benefit from having time to learn about yourself and people before entering into sexual activity that carries risks for your future life.

- Sexual activity and a relationship with a partner are complicated and require maturity to appreciate and manage.

- Sexuality throughout life has to fit within the framework of broader personal life goals and moral values.

- Good decisions in adolescence will increase your chances for a happy sexual life.

Fathers and Daughters

Whereas the suggested role for fathers in their son's sex education may seem somewhat "up-front" in tone, just the opposite may be most effective with a daughter. Your focus will not likely be on the mechanics of the sexual and reproductive system. One hopes that she will be getting this from her mother or another female caregiver, books, school, and so on. A father with sole custody, however, may need to provide all the basic sex information to his daughter or arrange for this.

What do you imagine will be your part in your daughter's sex education when she is ten or twelve or sixteen? Do you have in mind some information or messages that you already know you want to share with her? Folk wisdom has always told us that fathers worry a great deal about their daughter's coming of age and that they truly want to protect her from both physical and emotional risks. I have even heard young fathers, jokingly perhaps, talk about the benefits of arranged marriages for their daughter. This thought does reflect the sincere desire to help a daughter escape the sexual perils of today's world, but there are many more realistic ways for a father to influence his daughter's sexual development and decisions. While keeping in mind your own ideas on what you want your role to be, consider these as well.

You need to concentrate on building and maintaining a father-daughter relationship that is rich with positive feelings and messages. These can strengthen your daughter to meet the challenges of adolescence and young adulthood. Just as with a son, fathers cannot create something positive from a blank slate. A good relationship starts in childhood and results from time spent together on the routine activities of life—homework, chores, errands, sports, outings, shopping, cooking, home projects, hobbies, medical appointments, and so on.

Even with an existing solid relationship, fathers need to adapt to a teenage girl's changing needs and attitudes. Preoccupation with friends, need for privacy, and changing moods are normal, not a personal rejection of parents or family life. Adults with their greater emotional maturity are supposed to have the qualities of understanding, wisdom, and patience. Here are a few suggestions to help you stay involved, keep the relationship close, and support your daughter's healthy development.

1. Recognize her growing up with appropriate compliments not only on her appearance but also on her character, talents, and accomplishments. Keep these brief and simple, and ignore possible rebuffs or rebuttals. Do not tease or allow other family members to tease your daughter about growing up, appearance, weight, and so on.

2. Continue to offer to do things with her; give her rides to school or other activities; be aware of and ask about school, schedules, classes, homework, and the like. Don't back away from her life. Your steady presence can have a positive effect even if she never says thank you. I remember once, around the age of twelve or thirteen, walking through our small town with my dad on his way to work and feeling especially proud of growing up and my newly developing body. Even though my father hadn't said anything specifically about my appearance, I believe that my feelings came from knowing how much he valued and loved me.

3. Stay affectionate, in accord with your established style of exchanging affection, but accept her lead if she backs off somewhat. Don't take this as personal rejection or reason to cut off other forms of showing affection and love. Appropriate shows of affection are unique to each family. I have seen families in which teenage daughters were quite comfortable with continuing to plop themselves down on Dad's lap to talk, ask a favor, or just "bug" him a bit. Even adolescent sons who are not bound by male stereotypes are also known to do this on occasion with their moms, and although it is likely to come with humor, they no doubt also enjoy the closeness and affection that the moment allows.

4. Make a point to stay in the loop. Take an interest in and meet her friends (and boyfriends). If her extracurricular school interests or hobbies change, go with the flow. Offer to help with lessons, schedule arrangements, transportation, and so on. The more

you are available to her, the more likely you will have conversations where information flows comfortably between you, without your being the "inquiring mind." Staying in the loop makes it easy for you to know or ask about her life, friends, and activities without being too intrusive.

5. The heavy-duty conversations about feelings, dating, boys, relationships, sexual values, standards, marriage, and so on may or may not happen or come easily. You can do your part by tuning in to opportunities for offering personal insights, not by lecturing but by sharing certain selected situations and feelings from your own teen years or young adulthood or family history. You have to be in charge of maintaining your right to privacy, such as if she asks questions about your sexual behavior—although this seldom happens. But parents can appropriately talk about their own dating history, their family rules, their good and bad relationships. These moments let your daughter get to know you and let you show empathy for her stage of life.

6. With or without talking about intimacy and relationships, the way you live your life sends powerful messages. You model what love, commitment, and intimacy mean in a relationship by the way you treat your wife or committed partner. From this and your interactions with other women and men, your daughter learns the value she has as a woman and what to expect in a love relationship. From your involvement with family routines, child rearing, work, friends, extended family, and the community, she finds a model of marriage, intimate relationships, and family life. This point applies equally to sons and is another reason for parents to get their own sexual lives in order.

These suggestions do not imply a Pollyanna view of the father-daughter relationship—that it can be all sweetness and light. Naturally, there will be and should be family rules, routines, responsibilities, restrictions, and moral standards. These too are part of the relationship; they will come up for discussion and may cause disagreement.

In spite of differences, disagreements, or tense moments, continue to build the positive dimensions in the relationship (and remember that a good rule of thumb for any relationship is to aim for a ratio of five positive interactions for every negative). You will see that the parent communication skills discussed in later chapters can also help with conflicts.

———————

In this chapter, you took inventory of your own sexual hang-ups and the anxiety they might elicit in your role as sex educator for your child. You also learned that making changes to resolve your personal concerns can both improve your own sex life and increase your competence in dealing with your child's sexuality. As suggested earlier, don't be content to simply read and think about these issues. It is now essential that you take steps to make needed changes. Detailed directions for how to start are in Chapter One; go to the section "Taking Action: Changes, Solutions, Resolution" and start the process of change.

Many solutions for overcoming hang-ups are possible. If the characteristics of hypermasculinity and nonrelational sex have played a part in your sex life, reexamine whether these bring you happiness. Consider also how you will help your child deal with these same stereotypes that are so pervasive in our culture. If you berate or criticize yourself about your sexual history, strive to replace this judgment with more rational, balanced, or forgiving thoughts. If you discovered problems in your current sexual relationship, make a commitment to do things differently, make changes within yourself, and talk openly about your concerns with your partner.

Because some men hide painful emotions and personal problems from themselves and others, a good starting point is simply to talk about your concerns. Initiate a meaningful discussion with someone—for example, a close male friend, trusted clergy person, spouse or partner, physician, mental health professional, or professional who specializes in sexuality. Remember, you are not going to make needed changes overnight, but choose right now one concrete action and do it.

Another important step is necessary in preparing to become your child's sex educator and moral guide: learning to work together as a team with your child's mother or other caregivers, which includes clarifying your sexual values, beliefs, and standards.

3

Working Together as a Team

From the very beginning everything sexual should
be treated like everything else that is worth knowing
about. Above all, schools should not evade the task of
mentioning sexual matters.
    Sigmund Freud, "The Sexual Enlightenment of Children"

When it comes to your child's sex education, working together as a parental team is absolutely essential. Working together empowers parents and is the most efficient way to even the playing field; that is, it helps us feel that we adults are participants and in charge instead of helpless bystanders overwhelmed by the kids, the culture, or the burdens of family life.

Therefore, it's crucial to overcome the hang-ups that leave you feeling isolated and alone while you worry about your child's sexuality. "Her dad just can't handle the idea of her growing up." "My wife just doesn't understand boys." "The kid will feel like we're ganging up on him if we both keep talking about this sex stuff." "We just don't see eye to eye on sex." These kinds of thoughts divide parents just when they need each other the most.

Talking with a teammate is good practice for confronting your child's sexual concerns and questions. When both parents are working together and doing a good job, youngsters recognize and appreciate the fact that the adults in their lives care enough to give them accurate and consistent information and rules.

Who makes up the team depends on each family's structure and situation. Your role is to approach your partner—whether it be husband, wife, or anyone else who is sharing your life—and start talking about how you want to handle your child's sex education. A successful joint effort demands that you both understand the basics of human sexuality. You also need to understand whether any unique childhood characteristics put your child at risk of early or traumatic sexual experiences. Finally, you need to talk openly together about your hopes and dreams for your child's sexual future.

Regardless of the personal dynamics or even "bad blood" between parents or partners, you must work with these tensions and try to find ways to be a team. The two of you can decide whether one of you takes on a more active role or whether your roles should vary depending on the sex of the child. You can do a good job with your child's sex education even if the two of you take on different roles, levels of involvement, or ways of communicating. Disagreement on the major aspects of sexuality can be a problem, but if you know you disagree on some issues, you can then consciously plan on handling your differences in a way that benefits your child. Working together also means talking about your beliefs about sexuality. Ongoing talks about this subject will help you clarify for both of you the moral values and standards that you truly believe in and want for your child.

Benefits of a United Team

In most families, to have a united parental team focusing on a child's sex education would seem a rare phenomenon. Because of their sexual hang-ups, adults have accepted this situation as normal. This pattern must change, because it dilutes parents' power and puts them at a disadvantage.

Conditions of family life today make the team effort even more important. Married parents, busy with jobs and preoccupied with other family responsibilities, often mistakenly assume that they don't have to talk about how sex affects their child's life. And divorced parents, even if they don't have open conflicts, may not talk enough about issues that affect their child's welfare. Low-income families living in declining neighborhoods often face over-whelming odds trying to keep children safe, healthy, and able to withstand sexual risks. And even greater numbers of middle-income families are at risk due to the influence of peer pressure, the media, and the sexually oriented culture at large.

I recently heard a divorced father complain that when he told his daughter that age fourteen was too young to date, she replied, "Oh, well, Mom thinks it's OK, so she'll let me." In another family, a dad who overheard his wife use the word "vagina" in a conversation with their twelve-year-old daughter was shocked, and he later asked why she would use such a word in that way. Clearly, these parents should have been working together instead of being at odds with each other.

Leveling the Playing Field

Having a strong executive team can even the playing field for parents who feel helpless to influence their child's understanding of sex. Every day, your kids may be talking and hearing a lot more about sex than you. If you allow this to occur while you hang back in silence and denial, then you stay in a "down" position. Don't be a parent who fears that your child knows more about sex than you do.

The team approach forces the two of you to talk to each other about a lot of issues: your views and concerns about sex, the family's moral values, how you will guide your child, and so on. The action of talking openly with another adult and ending the silence opens up the many other benefits of teamwork. If you ever expect to replace your child's friends or the media as his or her number one information source about sex, you have to start with a united team.

Talking, learning, and planning with your partner provide another advantage. These activities are all essentially dress rehearsals for the actual performances you can expect with your child. Every aspect of teamwork enhances your knowledge, comfort level with sexual matters, and communication skills. From considering your differing ideas and opinions, you get hands-on experience with what you are likely to encounter with your child. Dealing with a team member prepares you to listen, ask questions, show respect, show compassion, be honest, offer to get more information, express ideas and opinions, reinforce family standards, and invite further discussions. When it comes to sex talks, these are the things that children want from parents.

What are other ways that a united parental team evens the playing field? Certain conditions of modern family life today seem to stack the odds against a child's having a healthy sexual future. The conditions described in the list that follows are linked to early sexual intercourse, which itself often brings immediate and ongoing sexual and life problems.[1] With a united team, a family can gain the energy and power to counteract these conditions and lessen the risks.

1. *Poverty and poor neighborhoods*. Low family income and despairing, dangerous neighborhoods mean fewer wholesome youth activities (such as sports, the arts, and hobbies) that build a child's self-esteem and foster positive life goals.

2. *Busy parents, busy children*. Middle-income families often experience the "do-it-all" syndrome and find themselves without the time or energy for talking, eating, and relaxing together as a family. With family members rushing off in different directions, parents may not have or use opportunities to explore a child's concerns about sex and growing up.

3. *Lack of parental support and supervision*. Parents' long work hours and their low energy when they *are* home may result in lack

of supervision, little supportive talk, and more coercive family exchanges, all of which are linked to teens' engaging in high-risk sexual behaviors.

4. *The power of peers.* Young people, especially males, who fill the physical and emotional emptiness of home life with a "family" of sexually active or risk-taking friends are more likely to engage in intercourse and sexual risk taking.

5. *The perils of mind-reading.* Generally, both teens and their parents have a poor track record in communicating clearly. In one study, mothers underestimated their sons' level of sexual activity, and sons underestimated their mothers' disapproval of their having sex.

6. *Risks associated with single-parent families.* Early first intercourse for boys is linked to mothers' having given birth as teens and having worked full-time when the child was five to fifteen years old. This research finding, however, may actually connect to overall conditions of poverty, such as a poor neighborhood, high negative peer influence, and few wholesome youth activities, as mentioned previously.

Parents facing these conditions are most in need of a united parental team. They often feel hopeless and cynical about being able to influence their child's sexual development and decisions. If you face any of these added burdens, teamwork will help you achieve the changes that may counteract them, such as the following:

- Gaining more clout than friends or the gang

- Finding and using the good elements in neighborhood life

- Coordinating work schedules to provide needed child care and supervision for your child

- Taking steps to get him or her into wholesome activities

- Talking openly about your hopes and dreams for your daughter or son

- Talking frequently about sexual risks and your family's standards

- Listening with openness, understanding, and respect in your talks about your child's life and difficulties

Capitalizing on Each Other's Strengths

With a teammate, you don't have to be superhuman—just willing to learn and grow. Between you, you can tap into the personal qualities that will help you both become the kind of "sexpert" your child needs. What characteristics allow parents to talk about intimate topics with their child when their gut screams "fight or flight"? Neither fight nor flight is an option if you intend to do your best to raise a sexually healthy child and young adult. So get ready to discover and cultivate the "right stuff" within you that will help you teach your child the "right stuff" about sex and morality.

There are several character strengths that I think are useful: courage, flexibility, endurance, self-awareness, a sense of timing, and commitment. The next paragraphs describe these qualities and tell why they are so important.

1. *Courage* is a quality that allows us to act and to do whatever is required, without withdrawal, in the most difficult circumstances: in a time of crisis; in the face of threat, fear, and anxiety; when life is hurting us or those we love; when sickness, loss, strife, or change upset our world. Think of your child's sexual development as a potential crisis—one about to happen at any point or actually even under way. "Crisis" is not an exaggeration considering the world that surrounds youth today. The wholesome "village" that used to help parents raise a child is no more. It has been replaced by an insidious consumer culture that trivializes and demeans sexuality. You need courage to face and combat this enemy and fight for your child's humanity.

2. *Flexibility* is a quality of good parenting. For example, when the family's needs change, parents often have to make adaptations that consider the goals of others—a partner, a spouse, a child, an aging parent. Flexibility has great value in dealing with your child's sexual concerns. It lets you "talk the talk" when the occasions present themselves, seize on the teachable moment, talk a lot or just a little according to the situation, try a new approach when others are not working, and be strict and firm when your child is young and more lenient about delegating responsibility a few years later.

3. *Endurance* is the ability to persist in a task and tolerate whatever pain and discomfort come with it. In modern life, emotional upset, not physical pain, is the common challenge. Endurance helps in talking with children about sexual matters, in either intense or repeated situations. For both parent and child, these discussions can trigger many different negative feelings: anxiety, awkwardness, embarrassment, worry, shame, and anger. Although by working through this book you may be able to eliminate some of these negative emotions or decrease their intensity, a certain amount of awkwardness or anxiety may still arise in discussing sexual matters. So endurance remains an essential quality to keep or develop.

4. To gain *self-awareness*, you need to monitor your feelings and behaviors, identify your needs, evaluate your progress, and examine yourself in the context of others. Whether this quality describes you or not, you can develop self-awareness by reading and interacting with this book. Talking about sex inevitably reminds us of our personal experiences. If we allow these memories and feelings to come to the surface, if we understand them, work with them, and resolve them, then we can take the giant step of separating our own sexuality from that of our child. With this boundary in place, we can have meaningful and sustained sexual dialogue with our child—again and again.

5. Because the need for sex education and moral guidance can arise at any moment, a *sense of timing* is essential for success. You

have to see the opportunities for teachable moments in your child's daily routine—bathing, dressing, grooming, shopping, cooking, doing chores and schoolwork, driving, reading, playing games, watching television, going through bedtime rituals. Just when you or they are busily involved, together or in close proximity, the questions or concerns often unexpectedly pop up. The challenge is to seize the moment, not miss a rich opportunity, know how much or how little to say or do, and recognize that your child's need to know is never likely to mesh with your preferred timing. The solution is to adapt to your child.

6. *Commitment* is a pledge or a promise not merely spoken but carried out with a substantial expenditure of personal energy. Parenting is a lifelong commitment, and most parents serve as nurturers, supporters, cheerleaders, buffers, and sounding boards for their children, right up to (and even through) adulthood. Now is the time to extend, in a conscious and planned way, all those roles toward helping your child grow into a sexually healthy and morally sound individual. Commitment enables you to follow through on good intentions to help your child with sexual matters.

Being part of a united team lets you capitalize on each other's different character strengths. If one of you falls short, the other can pick up the slack. You can also support and learn from each other. And don't forget that every chapter you read here aims to build the personal qualities and communication skills that will enable you to respond to your child's sexual concerns and questions.

Building the Parental Team

Now that you know the benefits, you are ready to form the team. Although parents often favor a united strategy in other parenting roles, they frequently ignore this approach to dealing with their child's sex education. For too long, one parent, usually the mother, has assumed independent responsibility for giving what little sex education children get.

A Team for All Families

Families differ in marital or relationship structure, social status, financial resources, access to information and services, and racial-ethnic heritage. Regardless of these differences, every parent needs a team. The simple act of asking a partner or others for help strengthens a family because it breaks the silence about sex education and creates a support network for learning together how to do the job.

Consider who will be on your team. Is your family headed by two married parents? Are you a separated or divorced parent? Are you and a committed partner living together as a family—whether straight, gay, or lesbian?

A divorced or remarried parent should, if possible, touch base with all the adults who coparent the child. The single parent (most often a mother) without a serious or committed partner can reach out to a trusted friend, relative, or clergy member with whom to talk about her child's sex education. Given her typical burdens of limited income, long work hours, and few social supports, the single mom need not face her child's sex education as just one more hardship to be endured alone.

The Ins and Outs of Recruitment

Recruitment is a step that most parents simply skip. Although they may worry about their child's sexuality, an even stronger emotion—some hang-up—keeps them from talking to each other about the subject. In other words, something holds them back. Most likely they fear rebuff or disagreement. Or worse, they don't want the partner's help or don't trust his or her judgment. Knowing the importance of a united team, you can learn more about taking this giant step of recruiting your teammate.

Asking for help and getting a partner to accept may be easy for some parents and not so for others. Given that all partners—married, divorced, and committed—usually have their share of communication difficulties around issues much less emotional than sex, some simple, down-to-earth guidelines may help.

Making Your Pitch No magical potion exists to guarantee success, and you are the expert on the best way to approach your child's parent or another person you want on your team. Nevertheless, you might find that the incremental approach of the recruitment ideas described here is useful with a partner who needs persuasion. Select ideas from the list and implement them in whatever order seems reasonable. Assume a positive attitude and stay in a good humor even if rebuffs come your way.

1. Mention that you are reading or have read this book, and let your partner know what it's about.

2. Don't expect or demand any particular response or action.

3. Ask your partner to take a look at this book, and leave it in a handy spot.

4. Share your reactions to specific parts.

5. Read passages aloud that you think are interesting.

6. Because sex is an emotional topic, allow for a variety of responses.

7. Listen thoughtfully and show empathy for your partner's responses.

8. Don't enter into any debates, arguments, or skirmishes over asking for help.

9. Allow time for the idea to take hold.

10. Share what you have learned about yourself and your own sexuality.

11. Show or mark a section that you think would be interesting, such as one of the personal inventories.

12. If your team member is also your spouse or sexual partner, you might talk about the book in general before bringing up any concerns regarding your overall relationship or your sexual relationship. (Chapters One and Two offer guidelines on how to do this, but the first step is to get your partner to help with your child's sex education. The personal inventories are just that and should come later, once your partner has agreed to help.)

Making Your Request When your partner begins to show interest, ask directly for help. In doing this, use the most basic communication skill, that of speaking for yourself. (This was mentioned in Chapter One as a tip for talking with your partner about your personal concerns about sex.) Although asking for your partner's help with your child's sex education is not as emotional as talking about your own sex life, there is a right way and a wrong way to make this request. Here are a few tips for doing it the right way.

1. Speak for yourself. This means using "I" statements to report your own thoughts and feelings and to make your request. Share your worries about this matter. Share something about your own sex education at some time during this conversation. This can make the point of why you want to do it differently with your own child.

2. Don't offer any mind-reading or judgments about how your partner will think, feel, or react to your request.

3. Make a point of listening closely to your partner. Ask specifically for his or her thoughts. This can keep the conversation going.

4. Keep the tone light and humorous if that is your style.

5. If the first attempt doesn't go well, end on a positive note, and consider using the incremental plan described in the preceding section.

Consider this possible way of starting the request: "I'd like us to work together on how we will deal with Chad's sex education. I suffered a lot from not getting any real sex education from my parents, and I want us to do better for Chad. Even though he is still young, I want us to be on the same wavelength in what we say and do and how we answer his questions and give him sexual information. The book says that if we are together on this from the time he is young, and if we have a plan, then it will be easier when he's twelve or fourteen. What do you think?"

Naturally, you need to make your request in a way that fits your family and your children's ages. If your son is ten or older, and you haven't done any sex education, then you can say that he is growing up fast, faces real sexual dangers, and needs his parents' help. It is never too late to get involved in this aspect of your child's life, though it can be more of a challenge starting afresh with a preteen or adolescent.

The Community as Team Partner

Because parents need all the help they can get, they should look for programs and resources in their community that are consistent with their goals for their child's sex education. Make a point of finding out if sex education programs or materials are available through the school system, your religious denomination, youth organizations, pediatricians or other health care services, community social service agencies, and government-sponsored public health programs.

School-based sex education programs are an immediate and accessible resource. Don't be content to simply sign the permission for your child to attend. Get specific details about the entire curriculum through all the grade levels, the materials used in classes, and the materials for parents. Use this knowledge to talk with your

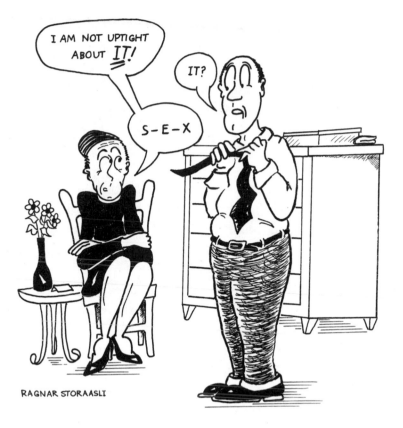

RAGNAR STORAASLI

child about what he or she is learning. School programs can serve as allies to all parents, but may be especially important for single parents. Take this same approach to find out what churches and other community programs offer to promote children's healthy and wholesome sexual development.

Parents often worry when their child does not have the constant presence of both parents in the home. They may wonder whether another adult as a role model might also help their youngster stay on a healthy track in life. Single moms especially often struggle with trying to be both mother and father. Besides recruiting a trusted, reliable team partner, mothers can also look to the community to help with her child's sexual and moral guidance.

General mentoring programs for "at-risk" youths have expanded in many communities during the past decade. A mentor is an adult who serves as a special friend to a child, with the specific role of listening, providing emotional support, tutoring, or engaging in enjoyable activities, all directed toward the goal of helping the child succeed in school, get a broader view of life and its opportunities, and develop short-term and long-term goals for personal growth, education, career, and life.[2]

Community resources for sexuality education do exist. To find out what's available, start by contacting the local United Way, Planned Parenthood, county and state health departments, hospitals and medical centers, universities, schools, and churches. Then check out specific programs and use those that are consistent with your plans for your child's sex education. If such programs are not in place, a next step is to learn why not and to work with other parents to ask for them. Make the community part of your team by finding and using existing resources or helping develop needed ones.

Team Training:
Sharing Knowledge, Purpose, and Vision

Parents who pledge to help their child with sexual matters at every step in life's journey go against a lifetime of conditioning that tells their body and mind, "Stop—don't go there." For you to change this overlearned knee-jerk reaction requires a conscious mental set to take on this mission in spite of the odds against it.

Because of the inclination to avoid the task, let others do it, or just hope for the best, you need preparation. Only prior training and practice will give the team the needed knowledge and skills to succeed. You cannot harbor the self-defeating notion that your child knows more about sex or speaks the language better than you do.

Training includes several levels. First, you gather "intelligence data" (basic and specialized sexuality knowledge). Next, you talk about the information and agree on how it applies to your child or family. The next level is even more personal: you discuss your hopes and dreams for your child's sexual future—not simply hopes to avoid sexual problems or tragedies but hopes for positive, healthy, morally sound sexual development at each childhood stage.

The idea of getting trained for this aspect of parenting is usually beyond the imagination of most adults. In talking to parents over many years, I have almost never heard them say that they had gotten a book on sex education, read an article, or asked advice on dealing with their child's sexuality. Once again, some kind of sexual hang-up kept these parents in the dark, unable even to find and use information that would help.

Every parent, no matter how smart or savvy about sex, needs training. Even the experts, myself included, can falter. Let me tell you a true story. It happened during the height of the Clinton-Lewinsky scandal, when the topic of oral sex claimed the airwaves. Sharon, who is a friend, fellow professional, and mother, actually faced and fielded the dreaded question about oral sex. Megan, Sharon's eight-year-old daughter with an inquiring mind, wanted to know.

MEGAN: Mom, what are they talking about when they talk about oral sex?

SHARON: Well, that's something that two people do to show their love and give each other pleasure.

MEGAN: But what is oral sex?

SHARON: It's a special way of kissing that two people do to show their love for each other.

MEGAN: How do they kiss?

SHARON: It's when you place your mouth on your partner's genitals.

MEGAN: So what did Monica Lewinsky do that everyone's talking about?

SHARON: She kissed the president's penis.

MEGAN: Oh, yuck. I'm never going to do that.

In recounting this story, Sharon admitted powerful feelings of anxiety and confusion. Fortunately, she had been giving her child appropriate sex education from an early age. Still, the nature of this question caught her off guard and left her feeling "awful" but determined to get through it. She said that she started off by trying to give general answers and avoid specifics, but that approach obviously didn't answer her daughter's questions. Then Sharon began to apply very consciously all of her professional training as a therapist and her clinical experience in working with sexual abuse and sexual dysfunction. She wanted to be "calm, open, and unperturbed," the way one is with clients, but "it was a whole different thing with my own child." A year later, in rethinking the situation, Sharon said, "To react with a good response to that kind of situation really takes training. It makes me think of the drills we did in lifeguard training. Over and over we practiced for the rescue, so we could actually do it, if needed, almost automatically. But as parents, we get no training to help kids understand sex."

Now you see why getting prepared with basic sexual facts and specialized sexual knowledge is so important. Because you have done the inventories in Chapters One and Two to help you face personal hang-ups, you are ready to keep learning about sexuality.

Basic Sexual Information: Obtaining and Using It

As you know, my purpose in this book is not to cover all the facts of sexual anatomy and physiology, sexual development, reproduction, pornography, and sexual problems and disorders. To boost your basic knowledge of sexuality, I offer many suggestions in "Sex Education Resources" in the Resources. I strongly suggest that you look for one or more of the up-to-date book titles listed there; they are grouped for parents and for children of different ages.

Start by buying one good book that covers major aspects of human sexuality. Having recommended titles ready to look up in a library or a bookstore will save you a lot of time. Bookstores sometimes put the sex education books for parents in the parenting section or even bury them among the books for children that deal with growing up. Ask immediately for help in locating the books that you want to look at, rather than filtering through the typically huge section on sexuality. (Most of these focus on improving your sex life. You can always come back to see if any of these might address your personal sexual concerns or problems.)

Take your time and look through several books before purchasing, making sure the book is up-to-date and comprehensive, has good diagrams, and uses other visual displays that aid in learning. It can be a comprehensive text on sexuality such as might be used in a college undergraduate course on sexuality. Or it can be one specifically designed for parents to bring them up to speed on sexual information that children need to know. Even the comprehensive books directed to teens are helpful, although I think parents should always have a more advanced book on sex than the ones they give their child.

Other sources for basic sexual facts include videos. These may focus on parents as sex educators or be directed to youth of different ages or to the family. The Resources list some examples and sources for renting or sometimes borrowing these without charge. (Video chain stores often offer these under their public service listings.) And consider some of the specialized Internet websites listed that address parental concerns about sex education, sexual information for youth, and teen problems associated with sexuality. In addition, check with your local school system for materials used in its sex education curriculum—for both children and parents.

Although this book is not comprehensive, it does provide considerable sexual information that boosts your knowledge. Throughout Part One, you learned about rigid gender-based stereotypes that are part of the sexual problems facing both young people and adults alike. These can affect a person's feelings about body image, attractiveness, sexual organs, sexual pleasure, and the meaning of relationships. Gender stereotypes put sons and daughters at risk for the same sexual problems that plague their parents. At some point you can use this knowledge with your child.

Part Two also expands knowledge about selected aspects of sexuality. Chapter Four covers the big sexual topics that young children need, though you should rely on other sources too. Chapter Five discusses how to teach six- to eleven-year-old children so that they expand their understanding of basic sexual facts and know what to expect during puberty. Chapter Six, which covers adolescence (ages twelve to seventeen), delineates the basic sexual information needed for youth in this age group (available in many books for parents and children) and covers in detail some important but typically neglected sexual topics, such as dating, relationships, sexual pleasure, and differences in male and female sexuality. These discussions offer specialized intelligence data that parents need but that are not typically available in a concise format to use with young people. The goal is for you to integrate this sexual information with the advice and moral guidelines that you want to pass on to your child. (The last section in this chapter will help you clarify your moral values about sexuality.) In this way, you use the material to help him or her think about decisions.

Specialized Knowledge: Children's Unique Characteristics and Risks

As adults and the architects of the family, parents are supposed to recognize and appreciate the uniqueness of their children. They quickly learn to adapt to a child's individual characteristics. Thus a parent might allow a baby who is by nature "quiet and self-sufficient" to remain in his crib on waking from his nap. That approach would not go over well for an "active" or "needy" child who begins shaking the crib and fretting the minute he opens his eyes.

Similarly, when it comes to sex education, the parental team should know about individual characteristics that create sexual risks, and help their child avoid them. For example, a child's early maturity, difficult personality, disability, lack of conformity to gender roles, and other traits cause fear and worry. But instead of learning, planning, and working together, parents often react with denial, helplessness, and open or covert conflict between them. They often then withdraw from each other just when they need to unite as a team to deal with the added risks. Whether these hang-ups are due to lack of knowledge or feelings of shame, blame, or hurt, parents need to overcome them, act like a team, and help their child with special needs.

Research has pointed to several characteristics that can increase the risk of sexual problems during both youth and adulthood. Having any single quality, such as those listed in this section, does not mean that the quality or condition *causes* the sexual problems. As suggested throughout this book, many interrelated conditions are linked to sexual outcomes. Still, if parents understand the qualities that create vulnerability, they can do their part to head off potential sexual risks and get their child on a healthy track. Here are several individual characteristics to note:

- Timing of physical maturity, and overall appearance

- Personality and temperament (especially tendencies toward excitement seeking, oppositional behavior, physical aggression, depression, and compulsive activity)

- Gay or lesbian sexual orientation

- Gender identity or role confusion

- Past childhood sexual abuse

- Disability (due to developmental delay and or deficit, chronic or acute illness, accident, and so on)

If your child has any of these qualities, he or she doesn't require kid-glove treatment, but you must give conscious attention to the timing, content, and emphasis of the sex education you provide. The brief discussions here explain the characteristics and risks and offer strategies for you to help reduce them. (Chapters Four through Six, which cover the childhood stages, teach the necessary skills for carrying out the strategies.)

Physical Maturity and Appearance Think for a minute about the age when you started pubertal growth and development of secondary sex characteristics. Were you on the early or late end of the continuum? Remember the responses of kids and adults toward the early maturers, both girls and boys. And what about the ones who were especially attractive at a young age: the "babes," the "hunks"? In answering these questions, you probably already know instinctively about the risks that research studies have reported:[3]

- Early maturity targets a youth as a potential dating or sexual partner and elicits interest from older teens or adults.

- Boys and girls who mature early have an earlier initiation into intimate sexual behaviors and intercourse.

- The higher testosterone levels that come with maturity are linked to initiation of sexual activity, especially for boys.

- Boys and girls who start dating at an early age, date often, and have a steady partner begin sexual intercourse at an earlier age than those who delay dating.

- Girls who date early (twelve to fourteen years) are more likely than boys to have first sexual intercourse during this age period.

The appropriate parental response to these risks will depend on many factors. Chaining sexy-looking twelve-year-olds to the basement wall is not an option! Clearly, the first important strategy has to do with the timing of the sex information. The child who is likely to mature early needs the basic developmental information *well before* the changes get under way. Second, sensitivity and support from you are critical, because the intensity of the younger child's emotions may exceed his or her cognitive ability to manage emotional reactions. Following these two guidelines, you should

1. Explain feelings of interest in and attraction to other persons and the many possible responses, positive and negative, that others might make.

2. Support the child's pride in growing up while also explaining that time is needed for him or her to become mature enough to handle intimate relationships and the risks of premature relationships.

3. Encourage the child to continue learning about sexual matters and to ask you about any new questions or worries.

4. Clearly express and discuss the family's moral standards and expectations with regard to sexuality and the child's total life, including rules and responsibilities.

5. Provide the support, care, and supervision that will enable your child to live by the family's standards and rules.

Personality Characteristics and Temperament   Contrary to popular belief, a child's personality and temperament are not permanently fixed and immutable, nor are these solely due to the child's "nature." Past, current, and future interactions with others (especially friends and parents) also are part of the "personality formula." Parents come to know that their responses to the child can either help modulate a given characteristic and channel it into a positive direction or exacerbate it and contribute to a negative chain reaction. Although you need not act as therapist to your kid, you must be savvy about how to deliver good communication, support, supervision, and creative ideas for problem solving.

Recent research on adolescents has linked certain personality characteristics and behavioral patterns to risky sexual activity.[4] Of concern are tendencies toward excitement seeking, oppositional behavior, physical aggression, depression, and compulsive patterns. Youths who have these qualities, compared to those who don't, appear more prone to make unwise sexual choices, as suggested in the findings listed here:

- Teens who value their independence, are more critical of society, and tolerate deviance are more likely to engage in early sexual intercourse.

- Boys who fight at school are at risk for early first sexual intercourse.

- So-called problem behaviors (delinquency, smoking, drug or alcohol use) are linked to sexual activity and pregnancy.

- Teens who take other health risks (alcohol or tobacco use, aggressive and reckless behavior) have greater numbers of sexual intercourse partners, a pattern that increases the risk of STDs.

- Girls who are depressed have more permissive sexual attitudes and associate with sexually active friends, factors that influence them to engage in sexual activity; however, girls' symptoms of depression are also linked to having more emotionally distant parents.

- Since about 8.5 percent of adult Internet users of sexual sites display some sexually compulsive tendencies and traits, it is possible that youth with obvious or extreme compulsive tendencies may also be at risk of developing unhealthy addictive behaviors, including in the realm of sexuality.

As early as possible in your child's life, you need to notice whether your child shows a tendency toward any of the aforementioned traits. At this stage, such characteristics may cause only minor problems that the family is able to manage. The goal should be to prevent such qualities from going into high gear during adolescence and driving the teen and family down dangerous roads. Thus the major parental strategy calls for a preemptive strike that aims to build and maintain a strong bond with the child, including respect for parental authority, good communication, and mutual problem solving. Within this framework, then, you should

1. Encourage and help your child discover and pursue appropriate positive youth activities that bring rewarding results.
2. Keep your child focused on achieving meaningful daily goals relating to school, home, family, and community responsibilities.
3. Listen and be responsive to your child's concerns and ideas so as to prevent feelings of alienation.
4. Clearly and frequently discuss the family's values, expectations, and rules.
5. Keep lines of communication open, but provide the involvement, support, and supervision that will enable your child to live by the expected standards.

Gay or Lesbian Sexual Orientation About one in ten young people struggles with concerns about sexual orientation. Homosexuality is not a personality disorder or psychiatric disturbance, but it does present challenges to the person going through the process of developing a gay or lesbian identity. Homosexuality appears to be a normal variation in sexual orientation that has existed throughout history and across cultures. Rather than resulting from any single cause, a person's unique sexual orientation—whether heterosexual, homosexual, or bisexual—most likely emerges from a complex interaction of several genetic, prenatal, developmental, familial, and environmental factors.

Some gay and lesbian adults have reported that they first became aware of their same-sex romantic interests in childhood, even as early as five or six years of age. More typically, the average age for this insight is thirteen for boys and fourteen to sixteen for girls. Awareness, however, is just the beginning stage in the process of developing a gay or lesbian identity. The majority of young persons struggling with this life task go through considerable mental turmoil before acknowledging their identity. On average, men arrive at this point around age nineteen or twenty, women at age twenty-one to twenty-three.

If your son or daughter is coming to terms with life as a gay or lesbian person, he or she faces special risks that you need to understand. If your child has concerns about sexual orientation, this understanding can help you offer the information, support, and guidance that your child will need. In addition, all parents have a duty to help all children gain an understanding of sexual orientation that will allow them to reject stereotypes, treat people as individuals, and avoid the hurtful practices of labeling and scapegoating people for being different.

Research studies have shown that many risks for gay and lesbian youths result from their confusion and isolation, much of which stems from society's negative stereotyped attitudes toward homosexuality.[5] The youth's reactions can then lead to further unhealthy emotions, thought patterns, and behaviors, including risky sexual choices.

- Young people's lack of information about homosexuality and their acceptance of negative societal stereotypes prolong their mental state of confusion and their devaluing themselves.

- To cope with feelings of differentness, teens may react in ways that delay their understanding, for example, consciously or unconsciously adopting stereotypical attitudes and behaviors associated with a heterosexual orientation, such as dating, putting down gays and lesbians, or assuming a stereotypical hyperfeminine or hypermasculine demeanor.

- Teens who do not hide their homosexual feelings are often subject to ridicule, rejection, harassment, and even violence from peers, friends, family, and society.

- Feelings of isolation and low self-esteem can lead to ineffective or destructive responses and behaviors, which create serious risks to teens' future lives: substance use, depression, dropping out of school, suicide attempts, alienation from family, and running away from home.

- Lacking self-esteem, a valued sexual identity, and good information about emotional and health risks, teens may make unwise choices about sexual relationships or activities, which leave them vulnerable to exploitation, STDs, HIV infection, and other personal, medical, and social problems.

Most gay and lesbian teens are afraid, and with good reason, to reveal their sexual orientation to parents. They want to avoid parental disbelief, disappointment, anger, rejection, or worse. In a sense, youths who keep their secret to protect the family from hurt take on the role of parenting their own parents. Putting the family's stability and welfare first leaves them to cope alone and without support.

Because having a gay or lesbian child doesn't figure in the dreams and hopes of most parents, facing that outcome typically sends the family into a state of shock and crisis. Still, parents should ask themselves whether the entire parenting responsibility has to break down under these circumstances. No one benefits if the whole family enters a conspiracy of denial and silence about a child's sexual orientation that goes on for years. During this time, they don't discuss it, seek information or help, or offer their child guidance and support. This approach comes close to a total abrogation of the parenting duty, something that would not happen with any other difficulty a child might face.

That such extreme reactions are fairly common suggests that parents truly struggle with this situation and need help. If you are in this situation, the primary parental strategy is for you to learn about sexual orientation and obtain support from professionals or self-help sources. (See "Organizations and Internet Information Sources" in the Resources for names and addresses.) The earlier this happens in your child's life, the better. The main goals are to prevent extreme denial and to enable you to become a source of support to your gay or lesbian child. You should

1. Obtain up-to-date information about sexual orientation from authoritative sources.

2. See a professional family counselor who is knowledgeable about sexual issues.

3. Contact the local chapter of groups that provide information and support for parents, such as Parents and Friends of Lesbians and Gays (P-FLAG).

4. Begin talking with your child, show love, and offer the support, sexual information, and moral guidance that can make your child's sexual life journey a healthy one.

5. Share the information with all family members to promote talk about feelings and to make healthy adaptations.

Gender Identity or Role Confusion Our culture still holds gender stereotypes regarding the attitudes, behaviors, and roles that are appropriate for boys and girls and men and women. During the past few decades, however, considerable flexibility in gender roles has emerged, especially with regard to careers, dress, interests, and family responsibilities. Many people now accept a range of sex-role behaviors both for themselves and others.

Gender identity is more than simply behaviors or roles. It refers to feeling comfortable with the gender that matches one's anatomical sex organs. Ordinarily, a boy with male sex organs identifies himself as a boy, and a girl with female sex organs identifies herself as a girl. Because most children are comfortable and happy with their gender identity, this rarely becomes a conscious issue, regardless of their choice of toys, playmates, or interests.

This type of clear and automatic congruence is absent when gender identity confusion becomes severe. In such cases, children are openly unhappy about their assigned sex and persistently reject it, saying that they *want to be* or insisting that they *are* the other sex. This level of severity raises concerns about the possibility of gender identity disorder.[6] Not merely a matter of behaving in a so-called tomboyish or sissy manner, this problem is "a profound disturbance of the normal sense of maleness or femaleness." The critical marker is that the child verbally disavows or expresses aversion to his or her assigned gender. In addition, the child may insist on wearing the normative clothing of the other sex, repudiate or try to hide sex organs, or want to get rid of them. One estimate suggests that gender identity disorder or lesser versions of it occur in 2 to 5 percent of children in the general population. Initial research and theoretical speculation suggest that a complex interaction of both biological and psychosocial factors contributes to the development of this condition.

A small percentage of individuals who have a strong sense that they have been "born into the wrong body" go forward with hormonal and surgical treatments that actually change their appearance and gender identity. Such individuals are often quite happy with this new identity and go on with their new lives with greater peace of mind.

Nevertheless, gender identity disorder as a diagnostic classification is controversial, even among health care professionals. One objection is that such a label reinforces society's rigid attitudes about gender. Simply knowing of such a diagnosis can increase parents' overreaction to a child who does not conform to stereotyped sex-role behaviors and lead to criticism or forced compliance, both of which are hurtful for the child. Thus an anxious parent might object to a child's play, games, or fantasies that include flexibility in sex roles. Another criticism is that parents will automatically look at gender identity or role variations as suggesting a homosexual or bisexual orientation, which is not usually the case.

Research suggests that several possible outcomes in adulthood are linked with gender identity confusion in childhood. If your child has this difficulty, you need to be aware of all these possible outcomes so that you can prepare to nurture him or her in whatever way best suits your child; competent professional counseling will likely play a role in any case.

- The majority of children with gender identity disorder do not continue to display the symptoms after puberty, and a minority of these youths seem to adopt a *hetero-sexual* erotic orientation.

- Some children with gender identity disorder adopt a *homosexual* erotic orientation (but gender confusion is not always present in the childhood of gay and lesbian adults, and nonconformity in gender role behaviors is not necessarily present in their adult lives either).

- For some children, the gender identity disorder continues through adulthood, along with the sense of feeling like the other sex, the desire to be and be treated as the other sex, and attempting to pass as the other sex.

Some such individuals go ahead and take steps to
change their appearance and anatomy, becoming the
gender with which they feel more comfortable.

A child with serious and sincere gender identity disturbance displays obvious symptoms that you cannot deny. These leave the child
and family vulnerable to public criticism, even ridicule, from family, friends, neighbors, and school personnel. In addition, the child's
remarks and behavior may elicit discord between you and your partner, including accusations, blame, and threats. Unfortunately, the
quality of your nurturance and discipline can take a nosedive,
adding to the child's distress. Under these conditions, the most
important strategy for you is to seek professional help in order to

1. Obtain a comprehensive assessment of your child's
   gender confusion, and guidance for dealing with day-to-
   day behaviors.
2. Resolve your relationship problems and disputes about
   your child.
3. Learn how to provide consistent nurturance, support, and
   love for your child.
4. Understand that the therapeutic intervention cannot
   shape your child toward a particular current or future sexual
   orientation.
5. Meet the child's needs for sex information and moral
   guidance at every stage of development and obtain further
   professional help as needed.
6. Stand by any child who, having reached a state of informed
   maturity and development, decides to make an actual change
   of gender.

Past Childhood Sexual Abuse The topic of sexual abuse in the lives
of children has emerged during the past two decades. Although all

studies of its prevalence have weaknesses, the findings overall are significant. A recent large and methodologically sound study asked questions allowing for broad interpretation of sexual abuse, including attempted or actual vaginal, oral, or anal intercourse; touching, grabbing, kissing, or rubbing against the individual in a way the person considered sexual abuse; and nude photos being taken of the individual or someone exposing himself or herself or performing a sexual act in the respondent's presence. The results showed that 27 percent of the women and 16 percent of the men surveyed reported a history of child abuse, with over one-third having not previously disclosed their abuse.[7]

Speaking generally, you clearly need knowledge of efforts to prevent abuse, ways to cope with the immediate crisis if abuse should occur, and additional steps to lessen any negative effects that might carry over to your child's future sexual life. The discussion here, however, explains the sexual risks for a child who has experienced prior sexual abuse and guides you in tailoring your child's sex education to address these risks.

Recent research suggests several areas of vulnerability for children with a history of sexual abuse.[8] These findings do not necessarily apply to all abuse situations, as individual experiences differ with regard to the intensity, duration, and damaging conditions of the abuse. Nonetheless, if you understand the general risks, you can be alert to troubling signs and symptoms. You can use this knowledge to better meet your child's ongoing need for appropriate sex education and to obtain special or professional help if needed.

- Child sexual abuse has been linked to such behaviors as persistent open masturbation, sexual preoccupation, and sexual advances or coercion toward other children.

- Child sexual abuse has been linked to such symptoms as fear, startle reactions, sleep disturbances, dissociation from reality, depression, and school and behavioral problems (although none of these is specific *only* to the condition of sexual abuse).

- Children who have experienced sexual abuse are vulnerable to further abuse, especially in cohabiting arrangements and stepfamilies.

- A minority of victims go on to abuse others sexually.

- Abused girls are more likely than girls who have not been abused to show such sexual problems as open and excessive masturbation, exposing their genitals, approaching adult and child strangers with hugging and kissing, and attempting to put objects into their genitals.

- Boys abused as adolescents are at risk of abusing other children, especially if they have lived in an unstable family situation or in a climate of family violence.

- Child sexual abuse has been linked to mental health problems and sexual dysfunction in later life.

Because each situation is different and a child's sexual abuse can have far-reaching effects for the child and family, professional help at the time of discovering the abuse is important to promoting a positive adjustment. A good therapeutic outcome should accomplish several goals that can make your job as sex educator easier. Ideally, your child would no longer have ongoing emotional and behavioral symptoms, and you and your child would be able to talk about the abuse when necessary and without avoidance, excessive anxiety, or other emotional reactions. The best parental strategy is to offer sex education and guidance that take into account the past abuse (when this seems relevant). For example, you should aim to

1. Convey in your talks the differences between normal, healthy sexuality and the child's experience of abuse.
2. Give special effort to help the child gain a positive view of healthy sexuality.

3. Tune in to the child's responses, behaviors, and goals for a sense of how he or she is progressing toward a healthy sexual identity.

4. Encourage further discussion about the specific ingredients of a healthy sexual relationship that is not abusive, and the qualities to look for in a partner.

5. Clearly convey the family's moral values, standards, expectations, and rules in the context of helping your child achieve a healthy sexual identity as well as prevent involvement in further abusive sexual situations.

Childhood Disability With regard to sexuality, perhaps the most important risk for a child with an *obvious* disability, regardless of its nature or cause, is that parents and society may deny the young person's sexuality. Such a stereotyped attitude ignores the individual's unique traits and abilities. Consequently, people with disabilities may receive little or no sex education and guidance and never gain the skills for understanding and managing their sexuality.

The discussion here focuses on one childhood disability, intellectual impairment, as an example of how disability can affect a child's sexuality and future life.[9] But the explanation is also relevant to other childhood health conditions, whether they are present from birth, the result of acute or chronic illness, or due to an accident. All children are sexual beings regardless of birth defects or other conditions that leave them with unusual physical characteristics or the need for special equipment such as wheelchairs, prostheses, or other devices.

As evident in the discussion here of intellectual or mental disability, children with any disability are particularly subject to certain attitudes that can prevent them from learning about sexuality and living a healthy sexual life.

- Society and parents often assign the quality of "innocence" to mentally disabled children and adults, regardless of ability, and assume they cannot or will not be sexual.

- Society and parents also often hold a contrary belief, namely, that the mentally disabled person has a strong sexual drive and lacks personal control.

- The mentally disabled child and adult are vulnerable to sexual exploitation and abuse by others.

- The mentally disabled child or adult who engages in public sexual behavior often receives harsher criticism, ostracism, and legal prosecution than an able person who displays the same behavior.

- Society and parents often look with disfavor on the prospect of intimate sexual relationships or marriage for mentally disabled persons, regardless of their unique capabilities or situation.

It is not possible to address guidelines or parental strategies that could apply to all types and degrees of impairment due to disabilities. One point is central: disability does not necessarily negate sexual interest and capacity. Sex education is essential to help the child gain, to the extent that his or her abilities allow, the skills to manage sexuality according to social norms. If your child has a disability, you will need to make adaptations to the usual approach to sex education, whether it comes from you or from agencies, special schools, or residential programs. Teaching methods must match the child's mental and physical abilities and will usually include much more than reading books and verbal discussion. Effective methods include using pictures, videos, and models of the body; letting the youth handle materials; demonstrating with role plays; and teaching skills step-by-step through the principles of behavior modification.

As parents of a child with a disability, you quickly learn that you must advocate for all the rights and services to which your child is entitled. Thus advocacy is the parental strategy of choice when it comes to a child's sexuality and right to sex education. Several steps are critical to this approach. You must

1. Become informed about sexual issues in regard to disability, especially your child's particular disability and prognosis.

2. Know what the service agencies offer in regard to sexuality education.

3. Advocate for and support effective and comprehensive sexuality education by the agencies that serve disabled children, youth, and adults.

4. Learn teaching skills from specialists and obtain effective sex education materials for use at home.

5. Arrange for your child to have continuing sex education throughout his or her various placements in educational, training, job, and living programs.

As is true for a child without a disability, you need not think that sex education is your total responsibility. You can draw on existing programs within the community, and if resources are lacking, you can educate others and advocate for sex education programs to assist disabled children in achieving a safe, healthy, and morally sound sexual life.

Sharing the Vision of Your Child's Sexual Future

Although parents often talk to each other about their child's day-to-day behaviors, achievements, and shortcomings, they probably don't openly share thoughts about their hopes and dreams for the child's sexual future. Future jobs, college plans, careers, hobbies, and talents—all these are acceptable topics, but the sexual future we want for our child is pretty much off-limits. At best, we worry alone or

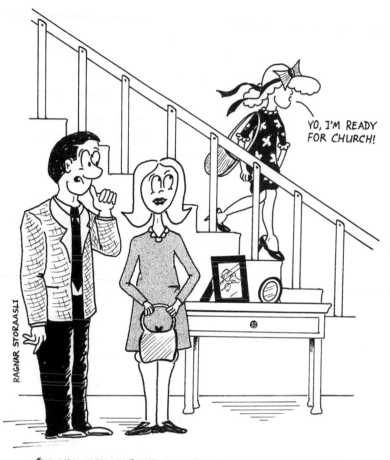

"DO YOU EVER GET THE FEELING THAT JOHNNY IS TRYING TO TELL US SOMETHING?"

mention the nightmares we hope will never come to pass—unwanted pregnancy, STD, early marriage, sexual assault, sexual offense.

Imagining Your Child's Sexual Future

If pushed, we may admit to a general hope for a happy marriage or a strong, loving relationship. Yet when we don't consciously think about what makes for a good sex life, we can hardly offer our child the tools for success. Even with the vague hope that our child will have a happy future love life, we have to admit that the odds are not good. Marriages for the current generation have a 50-50 chance of dissolution. And this figure is not likely to change, considering that kids today often draw their sexual values from sitcoms; "trash" talk shows; and movies, videos, music, the Internet, and a youth culture dominated by a mindless obsession with sex.

Maybe we cannot contemplate hopes for our child's sexual future because the outlook is so bleak. That is, we adopt a wait-and-see or hope-for-the-best mentality and take no action. Yet today and tomorrow are closely linked. We can overcome this hang-up by understanding that today's sex education will affect our child's adult life. Giving meaningful sex education and moral guidance "now" is our kids' best chance for a healthy sexual future.

Making a Commitment to Positive Hopes and Dreams

Imagine translating your highest hope for your child's sexual future into words. Would they go something like this? "I hope my adult child finds meaning and satisfaction in her total sexuality and comes to experience and sustain a loving, pleasurable intimate relationship. I hope her sexuality mostly brings a sense of inner harmony and spiritual wholeness and lets her feel a deep connection with her partner."

If these words capture some of your sentiments, then know that talking to kids about sexual pleasure, rewards, and meaning has to be part of sex education. The reluctance to do this is probably the central hang-up that blocks honest parent-child exchanges. Sexual pleasure is a difficult concept to talk about, but by the time you finish working through all of this book I think you will sense appropriate ways to do it and see how it fits with a young person's sex education. The idea of sexual pleasure need not be so scary if you consider all the family resources that can mold your child's sexuality: care, nurturance, protection, information, moral standards, family rules, supervision, goals, and preparation for good decision making.

Even parents who have achieved a good love and sex life often feel vestiges of embarrassment or shame about sexual pleasure. The feelings are probably much more painful for those who think they have failed at love and sex, are disappointed by meaningless sexual encounters or relationships, and have little hope of changing these outcomes. Chapters One and Two should have already helped you confront the hang-ups surrounding the idea of pleasure and meaning in your own sex life. Use your learning from those chapters to reaffirm the positive dimensions of sexuality. Then you can honestly tell your kids that the purpose of your guidance and information is to help them have a happy and meaningful love and sex life when they are ready for that life experience.

Eventually, sons and daughters have to negotiate their own path, and some struggle and pain are inevitable. What will help is an up-to-date road map that shows the best routes, the connecting highways, the targeted destinations, and the rest stops. As parents, you must provide this map. You can also share knowledge gained from your own past travels on the same road. In other words, you can offer an honest account of the sexual journey (including the pleasure, the risk, and the responsibility). You can also give advice on having a safe and rewarding trip (current sexual information and your views on the right and wrong of sexual activity). Then you must turn the wheel over to your child.

The best way that you can help a child toward a healthy sexual future is to know the markers of healthy sexual development during childhood. In this way, you have a sense of whether your child is on a good track. This is knowledge that both members of the parental team should have, because if you don't, you are likely to be at odds in your sex education efforts.

Personal Inventory

Characteristics of a Sexually Healthy Adolescent

This personal inventory is a listing of the markers or characteristics of a sexually healthy adolescent.[10] Consider this to be a verbal photo album that captures both the external behavior and internal life of a teenager.

Directions. Review each snapshot and think about it. Then go over it with your teammate as well. In this way you can begin to sort out exactly what your hopes and dreams are for your child's future. As you read each item on the list, ask yourself these questions:

1. Would I want my child to look like this picture at adolescence?
2. Do the ethical standards fit my religious or ethical values?
3. What would it take to get my adolescent to this point?
4. How do these characteristics apply to adulthood?

Self

Appreciates Own Body

_____ Understands pubertal change

_____ Views pubertal changes as normal

_____ Practices health-promoting behaviors, such as abstinence from alcohol and other drugs and undergoing regular checkups

Takes Responsibility for Own Behaviors

_____ Identifies own values

_____ Decides what is personally "right" and acts on these values

_____ Understands consequences of actions

_____ Understands that media messages can create unrealistic expectations related to sexuality and intimate relationships

_____ Is able to distinguish personal desires from that of the peer group

_____ Recognizes behavior that may be self-destructive and can seek help

Is Knowledgeable About Sexuality Issues

_____ Enjoys sexual feelings without necessarily acting on them

_____ Understands the consequences of sexual behaviors

_____ Makes personal decisions about masturbation consistent with personal values

_____ Makes personal decisions about sexual behaviors with a partner consistent with personal values

_____ Understands own gender identity

_____ Understands effect of gender role stereotypes and makes choices about appropriate roles for self

_____ Understands own sexual orientation

_____ Seeks further information about sexuality as needed

_____ Understands peer and cultural pressure to become sexually involved

_____ Accepts people with different values and experiences

Relationships with Parents and Family Members

Communicates Effectively with Family About Issues, Including Sexuality

_____ Maintains appropriate balance between family roles and responsibilities and growing need for independence

_____ Is able to negotiate with family on boundaries

_____ Respects rights of others

_____ Demonstrates respect for adults

Understands and Seeks Information About Parents' and Family's Values, and Considers Them in Developing Own Values

_____ Asks questions of parents and other trusted adults about sexual issues

_____ Can accept trusted adults' guidance about sexuality issues

_____ Tries to understand parental point of view

Peers

Interacts with Both Genders in Appropriate and Respectful Ways

_____ Communicates effectively with friends

_____ Has friendships with males and females

_____ Is able to form empathetic relationships

_____ Is able to identify and avoid exploitative relationships

_____ Understands and rejects sexual harassing behaviors

_____ Understands pressures to be popular and accepted and makes decisions consistent with own values

Romantic Partners

Expresses Love and Intimacy in Developmentally Appropriate Ways

_____ Believes that boys and girls have equal rights and responsibilities for love and sexual relationships

_____ Communicates desire not to engage in sexual behaviors and accepts refusals to engage in sexual behaviors

_____ Is able to distinguish between love and sexual attraction

_____ Seeks to understand and empathize with partner

Has the Skills to Evaluate Readiness for Mature Sexual Relationships

_____ Talks with a partner about sexual behaviors before they occur

_____ Is able to communicate and negotiate sexual limits

_____ Differentiates between low- and high-risk sexual behaviors

_____ If having intercourse, protects self and partner from unintended pregnancy and diseases through effective use of contraception and condoms and other safer sex practices

_____ Knows how to use and access the health care system, community agencies, religious institutions, and schools; seeks advice, information, and services as needed

At this point, review the list again. In front of each statement, indicate your agreement as follows: agree = plus sign (+); disagree = minus sign (–); uncertain = question mark (?).

Scoring. When you are finished, count your pluses, minuses, and question marks; you can enter your score here:

_____ Agree

_____ Disagree

_____ Uncertain

Only you can decide exactly what your scores mean. If you disagreed with or were uncertain about some of the items, ask yourself why. From reading the rest of the book, you may gain further insight into your reasons. If you wish, you can come back to this list again.

Being a Team Player: Dynamics, Disagreements, and Planning

Because families come in various forms, each parental team will have its unique structure and dynamics. No one family type "has it made" when it comes to a child's sex education. This aspect of parenting is an equal opportunity purveyor of confusion, worry, and trial-and-error learning.

The solution is to understand the dynamics of your family situation and the nature of your relationship with your partner. You and all the other adults responsible for your child's care must work within their unique life reality to offer your youngster the best help possible with sexual matters. For example, coordinating and planning can help overcome complications that arise from long-distance parenting, such as part-time custody or lengthy child visits during vacations or holidays. Gay and lesbian parents may need to pay attention to how societal prejudices might complicate their sex education efforts. And the single mother who has sole custody and responsibility for her child will likely use a teammate more for support than for her child's ongoing sex education.

All parents need to take an honest look at their unique family situation and the quality of their relationship with the team partner. You need to understand the differences between you and your partner and any special challenges you face in parenting. Take this step whether you are married and living with your child's parent, divorced and living in two different households, or living with a committed partner—straight, gay, or lesbian.

Different Strokes for Different Folks

Married partners often disagree on child care, discipline, and other aspects of family life that could easily affect the team effort in sex education. These are typical of complaints that I have heard:

> "My husband is too harsh with the kids, and wants strict obedience. So I find myself compensating for his attitude, being sensitive to their feelings, listening, compromising."

> "My wife wants our thirteen-year-old daughter to be popular. She buys her anything she wants—expensive makeup, clothes that are too old for her. She doesn't even listen to my opinions."

> "My husband sets no weekend curfew for our sixteen-year-old son. He's driving now, and all his dad says is, 'Call us if you're in trouble or need a ride.'"

Parents need to provide a reasonably consistent approach to the care, discipline, and supervision of children and to family rules, roles, and responsibilities. Although agreement in every aspect of family life is unlikely, differences in relation to such important issues as curfews, dating, and attending social events might greatly affect a child's sexual development.

Divorced parents also face challenges in building a strong executive team. Some findings about children from divorced families raise concerns.[11] Compared to youth from intact families, boys and girls from divorced families were found to be more likely to have intercourse at a younger age. Girls were more likely to have had a child before their first marriage and also during their teenage years. Another study found a link between mothers' dating behaviors and attitudes, young people's approval of premarital sex, and boys' increased sexual behavior. These studies don't mean that divorce per se causes these behaviors or that the family's divorced status is the critical link. Many conditions of family life could be involved. Still, if you are a divorced parent, whether a mother or father, you need to consider how your own separate parenting style might affect your child's sexuality and sex education.

If you and your spouse are divorced, reasonable questions to ask yourselves relate to the personal dynamics between the two of you: Do we criticize each other in front of our child? Do we complain about each other's discipline or supervision? Do we joke about or criticize each other's social or dating life? Are we giving our child both support and supervision? Do we inappropriately expose our child to our private love lives—either in talking about our intimate needs or in having noncommitted partners living in the home or prematurely involved in our child's life?

As these questions suggest, a divisive issue may be the different family atmosphere in each household. Ideally, parents would strive for a consistent approach to child care, discipline, and family routines and rules that affect their child. If you can't reach agreement or compromises, then the next step is to explain this reality in a straightforward, noncritical manner to the child. Children can adapt to different routines for each household if both parents give them the same message: expect these differences and follow the rules.

Some of the same barriers to creating a united team that I've already mentioned may also apply if you are a gay or lesbian parent. You too need to look at your family makeup and the parenting skills of the adults involved in your child's life. There is no research on whether gay and lesbian parents differ from other parents with regard to their child's sex education. You likely have the same kinds of hang-ups that hinder teamwork as other parents.

Additional personal and family stresses that gay and lesbian families face stem mostly from homophobia.[12] Society, your extended families, ex-spouse(s), and sometimes even the gay community may question the legitimacy of your family structure. Same-sex partners may also struggle with the demands of both the straight and gay worlds. In addition, you and your partner may differ about the degree of "passing" or "outness" you prefer in your own lives and relationship.

Ideally, when you and your partner tackle these issues as a team, you can strengthen your own intimate relationship. In the process, you likely become more effective in your overall parenting. For example, you will be better able to talk to your child about your family makeup to prepare them for possible negative reactions from others. As you might expect, adolescents, with their usual high need for peer approval, may need extra support from you to deal with this issue.

———————

Regardless of your family structure—married, divorced, gay or lesbian—a united parental team is good for all aspects of family life, but especially for your child's sex education. To become such a team, you and your partner need to look honestly at the personal dynamics between you. If tensions, conflicts, and stresses interfere with the team effort, you need to overcome them, find workable compromises, or prepare your child to expect and adapt to the differences between parents.

Disagreements

In spite of good effort, you may continue to disagree. The solution is to keep talking and to decide how important the differences are, given your child's age. For example, young children do better with clear and consistent messages about sexuality, just as they do with family rules and discipline. With older children, a possible compromise is to agree that one parent will have primary responsibility for the sexual topics they disagree about and the other will support that parent's approach.

If this solution is not an option, older children can understand that Mom and Dad may have different views on some matters. Both of you should be open about this and not pretend otherwise. You should also agree to respect and not undermine each other in your parent-child talks. You can say, "This is my view, but as you know, your mom [or dad] has a different idea." Too many areas of disagreement should be a signal that the two of you need to work harder on the basics, making sure that you have the same sexual information, share a similar vision for your child's future, and openly examine your moral values, as discussed at the end of this chapter.

Planning for Your Child's Sex Education

Beyond reading this book all the way through, doing the inventories and exercises, and talking together about these, you need only a few other immediate plans. These are the steps that will move you beyond simply thinking about dealing with your child's sex education and into action. Given most parents' poor track record on sex education, there is an obvious risk that you will swear to good intentions but continue to procrastinate. Get your teammate to agree on these follow-up plans.

1. Finish this book. Talk about the sexual content, strategies, and communication skills covered in the remaining chapters. Do the practice exercises with each other.

2. Decide whether you have any major areas of disagreement and agree to keep coming back to these to resolve them or find a compromise.

3. Decide who will obtain needed materials, such as a comprehensive book on sexuality, a sex education book suitable for your child's age, and so on.

4. Decide whether your child needs immediate or additional sex information—for example, if your child is a preteen who doesn't know what to expect at puberty, or a teen who is in a steady dating relationship.

5. Decide whether you will both be equally active in your child's sex education or whether one of you will take the lead. What will be the role of the supporting teammate? Decide whether roles will vary with a son or a daughter.

6. Instead of waiting for your child's questions, decide how you will take the initiative to provide sex education. Target a date and time for a first talk with your child.

Discovering Your Values and Moral Code

If you have ever seen one of the full-page newspaper ads promoting abstinence as the solution for the problems facing youth, you likely had an immediate emotional reaction. Maybe you felt a sense of relief, and thought "Yes, this is the answer. This makes sense." Or maybe you felt irritated, even angry, thinking that "just say no" doesn't begin to help young people understand and manage their sexuality in today's world.

My guess is that many parents feel something else: a sense of confusion. They don't see abstinence as a solution, but they also don't have a distinctly better idea for helping kids understand sexual morality. Uncertainty gives way to inaction. They put the paper away, decide not to decide, or figure they'll deal with it when they have to. This hang-up—confusion about sexual values and those that we want for our children—often keeps us at arm's length from their sex education.

But you can change that pattern. The final task for parental teammates is to resolve their moral confusion about sex so that they can offer clear values and moral standards to their child. Although the following brief discussion cannot do full justice to the topic of sexual morality, you can start by reviewing your beliefs and sentiments about sexual activity. Typically, these come from two major sources: religious or philosophical teachings and scientific knowledge.

Religion and Philosophy as Sources of Sexual Values

Consider your own religion (or other philosophy about life) and what it teaches about sexuality. Ask yourself some questions.

- Is my religion's view of sexuality primarily traditional and restrictive? (Usually, this means that sex is restricted to married persons, masturbation is wrong, reproduction is the primary purpose of human sexuality, homosexuality is not part of God's plan, a woman's interest in sexual pleasure detracts from her higher nature and role as wife, abortion can never be a morally right course of action, and so on.)

- Is my religion's view of sexuality primarily modern and human-centered? (Usually, this means that people can use their mind and conscience in deciding on standards of sexual morality, sexuality is part of being human, contraception can be wholesome and spiritual, homosexuality is likely an occasional normal variation in nature, the meaning of a sexual act depends on the human motives, standards of sexual conduct should be the same for men and women, a decision about abortion should be based on a woman's conscience and medical issues.)

- Do I agree with my or any religious perspective of sexuality 100 percent?

Science as a Source of Sexual Values

Science (which includes biology, medicine, public health, sociology, and psychology), through research, aims to describe "what is" and to arrive at principles about the way human life and the universe function. Ask yourself some questions.

- Do I accept some of the information and technology that science has contributed with regard to sexuality? (For example: sexual potential and interest increase at puberty; effective contraception and protection against STDs benefit people; most people have several intimate relationships in the process of seeking a permanent mate; modern societies encourage the delay of marriage; sexuality appears in various normal ways during each childhood stage; psychological reactions of love, lust, infatuation, and attachment are confusing;

people are not always clear or honest about their sexual needs and motives.)

- Do I accept some of the ethical implications of scientific knowledge about sexuality? (For example: people benefit from information about sexuality; knowledge of and access to contraception and protection should be available; responsible sexual decisions benefit both individuals and society; strict rules of abstinence and monogamy don't reflect how people in modern societies seek a meaningful relationship; divorce appears in most cultures, but stable marriages and intimate relationships benefit individuals and society; young people benefit from delaying sexual relationships to allow time for personal learning and maturity.)

- Do I agree with the findings and ethical implications of science 100 percent?

Applying Your Moral Values to Your Child's Sex Education

Beliefs about sexuality are only one example of values about life. For example, we also convey what we believe is worthwhile about education, health, economic security, marriage, friends, family life, and community involvement. Most people likely endorse sexual values derived from both scientific knowledge and various religious beliefs. Once you and your partner are clear on your beliefs, you can get practical about when and how to convey your beliefs and at what age your child can best understand which beliefs. Here are several guidelines to consider.

1. With younger children, keep moral explanations and expectations for their behavior simple. Some parents explain that sexual intercourse belongs in marriage (either believing this literally or using marriage figuratively as a concept that young children understand as meaning deep love and lifelong commitment).

2. For all ages, emphasize that maturity (age and emotional maturity) is necessary to make the important life decision whether or not to engage in sex with a partner.

3. To explain the deeper meanings of a sexual relationship, help your adolescent understand the nature of sexual desire, attraction, infatuation, and obsession. Talk about the possible risks and outcomes associated with such motives as curiosity, gaining status with peers, and pleasing or gaining a partner.

4. Help your child see the value of developing his or her own identity and some personal awareness before engaging in a sexual relationship.

5. Explain how partners need to be mature enough to talk about what sex means to each of them and to understand each other's needs and expectations.

6. Talk about why sex is likely to be more pleasurable if partners are honest, if they trust each other, and if they are capable of making a mature choice.

7. With older youth, explain your thoughts on the kind of relationship that is most likely to bring a satisfying, meaningful, and spiritual connection with one's partner.

If we as parents don't think about the deeper interpersonal meaning of sex and how we might want to convey this, we must remember that pop culture stands ready to tell our children why people engage in sex—perhaps as a game, a routine, an obligation, a happening, a pastime, a romantic interlude, or an evening's entertainment. Talking to your child about sexual values and morality is essential, and you and your partner should be clear on how you will do this.

When you and your partner decide to collaborate on your child's sex education, you take a basic principle of parenting—the united executive team—and use it to help your child reach a healthy sexual future. In doing so, you take a giant step toward changing yourselves, your family, society, and future generations.

Part II

Teaching Your Kids the Right Stuff
About Sex and Morality

4

Teaching Kids from One to Five

I hear in the chamber above me
The patter of little feet,
The sound of a door that is opened,
And voices soft and sweet.
　　Henry Wadsworth Longfellow, "The Children's Hour"

From the thoughtful look inward that you have just completed—thinking about your personal life, attitudes, and values about sexuality—it is time now to shift your focus outward toward your child. Your son or daughter is the reason that you have worked through Chapters One through Three. You put forth this effort to overcome your reluctance and ambivalence about sexual matters in order to take the lead in giving your child sexual information and moral guidance.

This chapter and the two that follow show you how to carry out this duty by addressing the typical sexual concerns and questions that are part of growing up. At each age level, children need sexual information and guidance that matches their emotional and mental development. If you provide this, layer by layer, year by year, you are giving your child a strong foundation of knowledge and morals that is crucial for coping with the tougher, more complicated sexual situations and decisions that come with puberty and adolescence.

This chapter offers you guidance on teaching kids in the youngest stage of life about sexuality. Whether you have a child in this age group or not, I believe you will gain much from this chapter. It explains the child's general emotional needs and the sexual information appropriate for young children. The sexual material and the parent communication skills are also applicable to older children, though in different forms. For example, if you didn't do much sex education with your child at this early stage, you may want to start with the simpler sexual information and materials presented in this chapter, even though your child is in the next age group.

You are likely to feel comfortable with the sexual issues that arise with very young children, although you may still feel embarrassment, or wonder if you are saying or doing the right thing. See if these questions elicit any memories or feelings:

- What was your reaction when your baby grabbed or touched his or her genital area?

- When your toddler was delightfully learning names for all body parts, did you teach the correct names for the external sexual organs?

- Did you also teach the names for the external genitals of the other sex?

- Did your child ask where babies come from?

- Did you obtain any sex education books designed for reading to a young child?

Whether your answers were based on memories of having already faced these issues or on imagined scenes still to come in your household, they may help you understand your current level of comfort and knowledge for dealing with sexual matters during this life stage.

Young children certainly don't bring the difficult sexual concerns that are typical of older youth, yet even the little ones can "push the envelope." This happens when a child *prematurely* (according to the parent's standards) raises a question or uses a sexual term that demands a parental response.

For example, Annie received a call from her five-year-old son's kindergarten teacher, who complained that little Allen had said to a girl in the class, "I want to have sex with you." Knowing that neither she nor her husband had ever used this expression in front of their son, Annie asked Allen what it meant. He replied that he didn't know, but he had heard it on television.

A remark such as Allen's definitely announces the need for some parent-child discussion about sex, but how much information to give is a legitimate question. What a young child needs at this stage goes beyond sexual facts, and parents have many roles to play in this process. This chapter

- Explains the emotional needs of young children and your role in meeting these

- Defines your role in teaching several basic facts about sex and morality for this age group

- Identifies important teachable moments, opportunities, and challenges

- Spells out parent communication and interaction skills that are effective with young children

- Offers exercises for practicing and perfecting these skills

Children in the "Cool Zone": Needs and Characteristics

Early childhood takes place in a "cool zone" with regard to a child's sexual concerns and potential to benefit from parents' sexual guidance. *Cool* refers to the more or less calm atmosphere surrounding possible parent-child interactions about sexual matters. This calm milieu exists for two reasons. First, because children from birth through five years old don't look sexual, their sexual gestures or questions usually don't set parental anxiety spiking as would the same behaviors from an older child. Second, young children are typically quite willing to receive information, guidance, and direction without challenging their parents' knowledge or wisdom. In this cool atmosphere, a great deal of sexual learning can and does take place for your child, whether or not you consciously plan for it. When you give good child care during this stage and explain a few basic facts about sexuality, you are building a strong foundation for your child's sex education.

With little ones up to about five years of age, we might see sex education in terms of answering such typical questions as, "Where do babies come from?" or "What are those big bumps on your chest?" Yet this early stage of development gives birth to more than childhood curiosities. Three major accomplishments are needed to get a young child on the road to a healthy sexual identity:

1. Development of a childhood conscience
2. A positive sense of his or her gender identity
3. Understanding of a few basic facts about sexuality and intimate relationships

We as parents obviously play a big role in whether our child achieves these tasks. Our most important contribution is a broad one: good parental care and nurturance.

Good Parental Care and Nurturance

Although it is simplistic and nearly a cliché, the best parenting advice is simple: remember that a child learns what he lives; providing good child care is essential to raising a good kid. Let's consider what this guideline means and how it affects a child's developing sexuality.

Parental care is central to a child's overall development. If care consists of love, kindness, and compassion, the infant and young child will thrive physically and emotionally. Child development theorist Erik Erikson has designated three tasks that the young child needs to achieve during this period; each indicates positive emotional growth. Specifically, he or she needs to gain a sense of *basic trust*, a sense of *autonomy*, and a sense of *initiative*.[1] These terms may seem rather abstract, but their meaning becomes apparent to any caregiver who regularly interacts with a child. We will take a closer look at each of these signposts of emotional growth, because they make possible the child's healthy sexual development as indicated by a childhood conscience, a positive sense of gender identity, and an understanding of a few basics about sexuality.

The child gains a sense of basic trust about self and the world from experiencing good care. Trust comes from having parents and caregivers who provide food, safety, shelter, and emotional security in a reasonably consistent and timely manner. These all come in a package through parents' feeding, holding, hugging, kissing, cuddling, soothing, nuzzling, talking, teaching, and generally tuning in to the child's needs and reactions. Predictable, loving child care lets the infant trust that the world is a safe place, a good place with good people. This sense of basic trust is the foundation for a healthy self and identity that will see the child through the rest of his or her life. This achievement also allows the child to trust parents' later guidance about sex and morality.

Having achieved a sense of basic trust, the child is ready to declare some independence from others and gain a sense of autonomy. More than merely the "no" stage or the terrible twos, this period finds the child intent on doing things by herself and asserting preferences, not simply needs. Just as parents tuned into the child's call for food and comfort, during this new stage they need to appreciate, support, and admire these independent strivings while also protecting the child from dangerous excesses. The toddler who senses that others respect her own growing skills will accept parental limits and guidance in various situations, including, for example, parental guidance on sexual values and standards.

Emerging around age four or five, the sense of initiative reflects the child's growing curiosity about the world and his place in it. He begins to have dreams and ideas about who he will be and what he will do. He may say that he wants to be a football player, be a daddy, or marry Mommy when he grows up. These and other fanciful stories reflect his unique spirit and call for parents and caregivers who will listen with love and attention. When others show empathy and appreciation for this desire to grow up, the child continues to believe in himself. With this foundation, he can then move toward more realistic personal life goals and dreams, such as those that strengthen adolescents as they make sexual choices and decisions. Teens who lack this sense of purpose often follow the path of instant gratification and set off on a sexual journey of "no return."

The Childhood Conscience

Good and bad, right and wrong—we expect a child to begin learning these concepts at an early age. Parents readily recognize that the childhood conscience has a lot to do with sexuality, but they may not know just how early it begins to form and that children learn right and wrong from the way others treat them.

The sense of trust, autonomy, and initiative forms the bedrock foundation for the child's developing conscience. Trust in the goodness of parents and the world lets children see themselves as good and valuable. From a parent's empathy for the child's desire to be independent and grown up, the child learns also how to identify with the feelings of another person. Even infants are capable of a sympathetic response to the distress of someone in their presence. Parents can also specifically teach the toddler or older child to pay attention to the pain of others and offer help. Empathy is part of teaching a child how to behave in a grocery story, a restaurant, or at Grandma's house. As he learns to behave in ways that consider another person's feelings, the child begins to see the other person as a subject, as someone who is just as important as he is. Empathy is necessary for the child to truly understand the Golden Rule, which is central to the childhood conscience: treat others as you wish to be treated.

The next component in the childhood conscience is the moral compass that helps the child choose and act on the right behavior. Out of her sense of right and wrong, her attachment to parents, and their direct guidance, a child naturally strives to live by rules. Once again parental care and nurturance enter the picture. The young child's motivation to follow the moral compass at this early stage and to "do the right thing" derives from love of parents, acceptance of their authority, and need for their approval.

If a child does not develop a conscience during this early stage, the facts about sexuality will simply pass into a moral vacuum. This is why parents need to give their child good care and nurture the developing conscience. What exactly can you do to help your child gain this early basis of knowing right and wrong? Your day-to-day care, talking, teaching, and modeling help your child develop the following qualities that serve as a basis for the conscience:

- Awareness of his or her own feelings and ability to express them

- Love and valuing of himself or herself

- Increasing self-control in situations that demand it

- Awareness of others and ability to read their emotions

- Caring feelings and gestures toward others

- Decisions and behaviors that reflect fairness to others

A child must begin learning at a very young age what it means to be a human being and how to live by the rules of society. Without this broad moral foundation, specific sexual values and guidelines on sexual conduct will have little meaning. Avoiding sexual risks, valuing a partner, protection of self and partner, abstinence, personal self-control, and responsibility—these sexual standards will have no meaning for an eleven-year-old who has never developed a childhood conscience.

Positive Sense of Gender Identity

Typically by the age of two, the child has a clear sense of his or her gender identity, and parents play a part in making sure that the child also feels positive about being a boy or being a girl. They help by teaching the names for the child's sexual organs and for those of the other sex, by explaining how and why boys' and girls' bodies differ, and by affirming that each has just the right equipment. This simple approach shows acceptance of the child's gender and of sexuality as a routine, normal part of life—not denied, not secret, not shameful.

As suggested in earlier chapters, rigid prescriptions for how boys and girls should behave are central to many of the problems that teens and adults experience in intimate relationships. Although gender affects everyone and is bound to influence child rearing, you can do your children a favor by monitoring your own unconscious, automatic gender-biased responses. These often come out in such phrases as "Boys don't . . ." or "Girls don't . . ." or, worse, in the use of hurtful terms such as "sissy" or "crybaby."

You should also be alert to knee-jerk responses that label or criticize a child's interests or play according to stereotyped notions of masculine or feminine. The conditions of today's world in terms of jobs, careers, and family life have departed considerably from roles dictated by rigid gender stereotypes.

We need to prepare children for the real world by giving similar, nongendered messages to both boys and girls about the benefits of physical play and strong bodies, their achievements, their unique interests and talents, their sensitivity and thoughtfulness toward others, their help with family routines, and their value as a whole person. Girls need to gain a sense of personal value that goes beyond physical appearance and being a sex object. Boys need a sense of masculine identity that encompasses deep sentiments of caring, compassion, and commitment. Loosening the constraints of gender stereotypes is a way to help children grow up to feel good about themselves. This strength will help them combat the continuing onslaught of gender bias and teasing that can attack self-esteem at puberty and adolescence.

Understanding of a Few Basic Sexual Facts

The nature of early childhood and a child's experience in the world naturally suggest several basic facts about sexuality that youngsters need to know. Kids see and touch their bodies and sexual organs. They learn toilet habits. They learn to bathe, groom, and dress. They notice the bodies and sexual organs of others, either at home or in day care. They may consciously explore sexual organs through "playing doctor." They see pregnant women or new babies. They see models of marriage or love relationships. All these experiences give rise to sexual questions and to opportunities for parents to explain a few basic sexual facts.

There are relatively few sexual topics that young children need to know or are likely to ask about. When your child is between the ages of about three to six, you should expect to field questions or respond to behaviors that have to do with the following sex-related issues: naming and explaining the sexual organs, touching, toilet training, masturbation, nudity, body safety, playing doctor, where babies come from, and obscene words. When your child is at this stage of development, you are in a position to have considerable control over what and how your child learns about these sexual topics. And because questions usually arise in the context of family life, your being prepared for this central role is the best course of action.

Before learning about exactly how you can address these basic topics (which is covered in the next section), keep in mind that these parent-child talks provide the child with more than an understanding of some sexual facts—they reveal whether you are an "askable" parent. The young child's level of curiosity and understanding will be limited, so don't expect to give out a great deal of information for a single question. Because of their limited mental development, young children will need further explanations, may forget information, and may ask the same questions again—which is why you must be willing to listen and answer. That response lets your child know that you are a parent who will answer any kind of question, has wisdom and authority, and can be trusted. When you calmly and thoughtfully answer all questions, however briefly, your child learns that he or she can come back again and again with questions.

The Role of Parents in Teaching About Sex and Morality

Most, but not all, young children will ask about at least some of the topics mentioned earlier. Your own willingness to tune into your child's sexual concerns may be a factor in whether he or she asks about sex. You can become more comfortable with the prospect of these questions by remembering characteristics of the young child. Don't expect to give a great number of technical details. Keep interactions brief to match a young child's attention span, and listen closely and explore for what your child is really asking. It's always a good idea to offer praise for asking the question and then determine your child's understanding—for example: "That's a good question. What do you think sex means?" or "Where do you think babies come from?"

For the child who hasn't asked sex-related questions by age five, consider reading a book with your child that explains simple sexual facts in engaging ways that match the learning ability of this young age. I strongly advise having such a book on hand. In this way you are prepared for the questions that come or for taking the initiative to explain some basics about sex accurately and according to your preferred timing and moral viewpoint.

Many parents are not aware of children's books about sexuality. To learn more about these, browse through the children's, juvenile, teen, and personal growth sections of bookstores. Or ask for assistance in locating children's books that deal with sexual topics. Take time to look closely at choices, decide which ones fit your values, and consider how you can add your unique moral perspective. You might also obtain resource lists from your religious denomination. Check your local libraries for titles that you might want to borrow instead of purchase. (See "Sex Education Resources" in the Resources for complete details about books mentioned in this and other chapters.)

In answering a child's questions or reading a book together, make a point of offering accurate information in a matter-of-fact manner, just as you would in teaching your child about other aspects of life, such as food, clothing, playing, games, shopping, safety, and so on. Seeing the situation in this way enables you to be calm, positive, thoughtful, and supportive. In response to a child's questions or a sexual situation, avoid gestures and words that convey shock, shame, disgust, anger, or personal teasing. In addition to giving the facts, you can also explain your moral viewpoint if this seems to apply to the situation.

Recently, I heard a story about how the typical routine of bath time led to an unexpected question from a child. Barb, a conscientious mother, was supervising six-year-old Ben's bath when she handed him the soap and reminded him to wash his penis (a term she had just started to use, instead of "privates," after reading an article on sex education). With that, the following conversation took place.

BEN: Bonnie [an eight-year-old playmate] found one of these outside.

MOM: Found a penis outside?

BEN: No, what you put on one.

MOM: You mean she found a condom?

BEN: Yeah, I guess.

MOM: Kind of like a plastic, rubber thing?

BEN: Sort of like a little bag.

MOM: You mean a condom?

BEN: I guess.

MOM: You know what that's for?

BEN: No.

MOM: You shouldn't touch something like that, stuff you find on the street. It's dirty.

Here we see Barb calmly keeping the conversation going, clarifying what her son meant, and using accurate terms. She decided that she did not need to explain the use of condoms, but connected the situation to other learning she wanted her child to remember, namely, not to handle dirty stuff from the street. She did all this without shaming him for asking or criticizing his playmate for showing him the condom. Another parent might have chosen to offer further information. We see here how the normal routines in Ben's life, playing and bath time, gave way to this brief talk; this is but one example of how children's everyday experiences growing up create opportunities for parents to explain several basic facts about sex.

Naming and Explaining Sexual Organs

When a toddler is learning the names for his or her body parts, this is the time to include proper names for the sexual organs. Simple naming of the external sexual organs is usually all that is necessary at this stage—vulva, penis, scrotum—because these are what are visible. Once your child knows the names, you can then continue to use the terms comfortably and matter-of-factly as future sexual situations or questions arise, such as during bath time or during a doctor's visit. You should also offer the names for sexual organs of

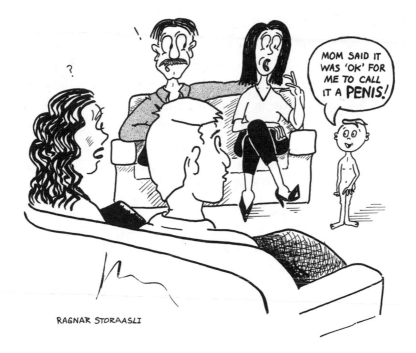

RAGNAR STORAASLI

the other sex, explain that both boys and girls have just the equipment they need, and mention that other kids or adults may use
other informal terms.

You may also add your moral or ethical view as well. For example, "God gave us our wonderful bodies, and we must take good care
of them," or "Our bodies let us do so many things—run, jump, play,
learn, have fun, enjoy life." As the child reaches age five or six,
some additional brief explanation of the function of the sexual
organs may be appropriate, such as on the topic of where babies
come from.

Touching

Infants and toddlers naturally explore and touch their sexual organs.
This is part of their learning and exploring everything around them,
and the body is the basic starting point. Babies initially touch the
entire body in a random manner, but they also learn that touching

the genital area brings pleasurable sensations. Touch is one of the senses, and learning about it is part of healthy emotional development. The child is becoming aware of his or her body as separate from, yet connected to, the rest of the world. Enjoying the feel of walking barefoot in the grass, the heat from the fireplace, the scalp massage during a shampoo—all these experiences and many more are the stuff of sensual learning. If you can see a baby or toddler's body exploration in this way, you won't automatically scold or take the child's hands away if they should settle on the genital area.

Toilet Training

Toilet training and explaining the body's processes of elimination call for calmness and a mature, rational attitude from you. Toilet training too is a learning experience for the child, and you need to focus on accomplishments each step of the way. Look for the chance to reward and praise even the smallest behavior in the right direction, for example, just sitting on the potty for a couple of minutes whether or not a production takes place. Monitor your own obsessiveness and annoyance. Accidents are inevitable, and shaming a child is very hurtful. Because the sexual organs are linked with elimination, be sensible in teaching habits of cleanliness, and avoid emotional words like "dirty," "nasty," and so on.

Masturbation

Some young children, but not all, may engage in more focused touching or self-stimulation because it creates pleasurable sensations. The challenge is to see this as a normal part of learning and not as some deviant behavior. Because of taboos surrounding masturbation or because of their own unresolved shame about it, parents often have an automatic gut reaction that such touching is just "not right." With effort, you can recover from this initial reaction and calmly explain, "Touching your sexual organs is something you do in private." Depending on your viewpoint and comfort, you might add a remark such as, "I know that feels good, but remember what I was explaining about public and private. . . ." Privacy is an important concept that will continually come up with many sexual matters.

Nudity

Parents often have questions about nudity within their own home. No one gets too concerned with the toddler who finishes bath time by running naked into the living room or even outdoors. This is more like a game, and most parents handle it this way. The same applies if the child decides to strip in front of others or after swimming. A simple reminder about privacy and clothes in public places is all that's needed. But parents wonder about letting a child see them nude, such as in the process of showering or dressing. On this matter, you need to determine your own comfort level and beliefs about nudity. If you prefer privacy, simply close the door and explain this to the child. Even if you have been comfortable being nude in front of your child from infancy on, you will still need to be sensitive to changing reactions, especially with an opposite-sex child or one who is overly inquisitive about genitals.

Children's needs change, and around age five and six most youngsters develop a sense of modesty and want and ask for privacy. You should respect the importance of private boundaries—your own and your child's. All family members should have a say in who sees their bodies. When children reach this point, knocking on closed doors should be a rule for the whole family. Bathing young siblings of the opposite sex together is typical for many families. This too needs to change as children start approaching age five or six if they want to bathe alone, if they focus excessively on sexual organs or questions about them, or when you think it advisable.

Nudity and privacy are more complicated in the case of remarriage or cohabiting arrangements, which may also include live-in or visiting stepsiblings. You should be sensitive to the need for new rules regarding nudity, bathing, grooming, shows of affection, and privacy. The biological parent should take the initiative to bring up and clarify these matters, without waiting for a family crisis to happen. Children should have their say, and everyone should understand and agree on clear family rules. The lack of clear personal boundaries often results in their violation, causing problems in newly formed families that can range from complaints and arguments to allegations of sexual abuse.

Body Safety

The past ten to fifteen years have brought increased public awareness about child sexual abuse. Most parents will have heard about the importance of teaching young children to protect themselves from possible sexual molestation or assault by older children or adults. Programs that teach the simple concepts of "good touch, bad touch" are common in preschools, kindergarten, and early elementary grades. You should make sure that what you and your child's school teach about body safety presents a balanced view and does not create an atmosphere of fear, danger, or shame around sexuality. I have heard of a young child coming home from such a school program and question whether it was OK for Daddy to dry her off with a towel after a bath.

Before learning to protect private boundaries, children should have gained a positive sense of their own sexuality and sexual organs. Parents who follow the guidelines described earlier for teaching simple sexual facts will convey that sexuality is a normal part of human beings. This positive understanding is a good foundation for continuing to explain that the child owns his or her body, can touch it, and has a say in who else touches it. Parents and educators make a serious mistake if the child's first open discussion of or naming of sexual organs takes place in the context of information or warnings about body safety.

By preschool age (about three years old), the typical child can understand the idea of body safety. Children can learn at this point that only they, their parents during bath time, or a medical person doing an examination can touch their private parts. It is also important to teach them how to refuse an inappropriate touch, that it is OK to tell if this occurs, and that it's not the child's fault if it does happen. Reminders are important, especially during times of transition, such as a divorce, custody changes, a parent's new marriage, or going to camp or a new school.

You should gauge your child's response to this information to decide the amount of time and detail needed and to watch for signs of worry or fear. Answer any questions and mention that you will talk more about this matter again or whenever new questions come up. Such talks should take place in a calm, matter-of-fact tone, and not right before a child's bedtime or departure from home.

Playing Doctor

Playing doctor is an activity that children may do out of normal curiosity to learn about and see sexual organs, especially of the opposite sex. With young children who are *similar in age*, you may calmly stop the activity, say nothing to shame the children, and offer to read again the child's book of sexual information that teaches about the body. This activity should not be used as an example of inappropriate or "bad touch." If it happens often or as your child gets older, you should explore for reasons and continue to talk about keeping sexual organs private.

Where Babies Come From

Nearly every preschooler will ask and needs to know where babies come from and how they develop. This question often upsets parents because they instantly think about the adult perspective of intercourse. Once again, I strongly advise you to obtain children's books that give brief, general, but accurate information on this and other sexual topics. Such books, especially those that reflect a family's moral values, help alleviate concern about what words to use and how much detail to give. They are also visually appealing with colorful or humorous illustrations that engage children's interest.

Several books designed for toddlers focus simply on pregnancy and how the baby develops, without mentioning the act of intercourse as the means for bringing egg and sperm together (for example, *Look How a Baby Grows, How Are Babies Made?* and *The Miracle of Life*). This type of book offers an excellent starting point for teaching about sexuality from a very early age and gets you in the habit of reading to and with your child about sexual topics. For the older child, other books include simple but accurate accounts of intercourse. (A classic example is Peter Mayle's *Where Did I Come From?*) You should prepare for the inevitable question of how the baby gets started in the first place. Typically by the age of five, the child will need to know these general sexual facts about the way that babies come into the world:

- A special way that a husband and wife (or man and woman) show their love is when the man puts his penis in the woman's vagina.

- If they decide to, they can make a baby this way.

- The baby grows in a special place in the mother's body, not the stomach where food goes.

- When the baby is fully developed, it comes out through the mother's vagina.

- The new mother's breasts produce milk, so the baby may nurse at the breast or through a bottle or both.

An explanation that includes these few general but accurate facts can accomplish many goals. It can link pregnancy to several ethical standards that deal with adulthood, marriage, love, and choice. It can prevent common childhood myths, such as thinking that parents simply get (buy?) a baby from the hospital. If they haven't heard an explanation, some children think the baby is in the mother's stomach, where it gets food to grow, and will come out of the anus just as in the elimination of body waste.

Regardless of the account of intercourse in a children's book, you can add or emphasize the exact moral values you want to convey, such as choosing whether to use the terms "husband and wife" or "man and woman." In language a young child can understand, you may further link intercourse and conception to your religious or philosophical beliefs. When you have included your moral view on the purpose of intercourse and conception, you are in a good position to handle the inevitable later situations involving "four-letter words" or other street terms for intercourse. You will also have a good base for adding further details about these facts as your child gets older or asks more questions—for example, "Remember when we talked about where babies come from and the mother's egg and the daddy's sperm? Now that you're older, you're ready to learn more about this wonderful story of how a baby grows."

A simple account of adult intercourse also achieves another important goal. It adds balance to any discussion about inappropriate touch and body protection. It lets a child see that adults can choose to let another person see and touch their private parts. This points up the importance of giving young children all of the basic facts we've covered in this chapter. From the various factual explanations, they get a balanced view of sexuality, they learn that sexuality is part of life, they need not make up their own myths to explain sexual organs or pregnancy, and they learn to trust that parents are a good source of information.

Obscene or Slang Words

Parents may have different views about which slang or obscene words they do not want their child to use. Usually we give little thought to this until our child blurts out an offensive word in our presence or in public. With young children, most parents know the standards they want and quickly act to deal with the situation. Sex educators agree that some thought as well as a calm attitude should go into your explanation. First, you might ask where the child has heard a particular word and what he or she thinks it means. Then explain, in simple terms for a young child, what the word means and why you object to it—for example, it aims to show anger by denigrating a person or portraying a sexual act or body part as degrading, or it aims to shock people, or it is inappropriate in certain situations, or all of these.

Sex educators often suggest that the parent use the objectionable word at least once in the explanation. Showing that you know the word and can use it in your talk reduces the chance that your child will use it again simply to get an emotional reaction from you. Finally, check out whether your child has understood your reasoning, and then give the rules that you expect your son or daughter to follow.

———————

A final important point is that most young children will not remember the details about sexual information you give on the big topics, so they may ask the questions again. Even with good explanations, your child may still reveal confusion about how a baby grows or gets started, or about other sexual facts. These are complicated processes, and the young child's cognitive abilities are still developing. Expect to follow up with further talks and rereading of the same books or more advanced ones through the years.

Teachable Moments, Opportunities, and Challenges

Your child's first five years of life offer you many venues for teaching him or her about sexuality. This is because early childhood development centers on the child's learning about self, others, and the rules of human life. As mentioned earlier, this learning is embedded in good child care, which lays the foundation for the development of the childhood conscience and a positive sense of gender identity. As a parent, you promote these important milestones through all of your interactions and teachings with the child. In other words, every time you teach your child about general life values and right conduct, you are adding building blocks to the conscience, which will be essential for understanding moral values and standards for sexuality.

Teachable Moments and Opportunities

Even in explaining the few basic facts of sexuality, you need not look too hard for specific teaching opportunities, as these readily arise in the child's everyday activities. You will see situations that call for brief explanations of sexual facts if you are alert to all the things the child is learning—the names of body parts, bathing, grooming, toileting, dressing, playing with others, conduct with adults and playmates, and so on. You can also offer lessons about sex, love, and life in response to the child's remarks or questions and to images and situations that the child sees on television or in movies.

In addition to the naturally occurring opportunities, you can also take the initiative to provide basic sexual facts and general moral guidance. Although most young children will ask sexual questions, you need not wait for inquiries. I cannot emphasize enough the importance of children's sex education books. Take time to select and read to your child from books that provide simple but accurate explanations of sexual facts. If reading together is a family routine (and it should be!), children will accept books on sexual topics as a normal, enjoyable way to learn. With an early start, your child will comfortably read such material with you through middle childhood or even later. Remember that you readily buy books and stories that teach your child about the world and lessons about life. So make it a point to obtain sex education books as well and to select those that reflect your religious or ethical beliefs.

Another area in which you can take a proactive role relates to television images or situations that can serve as a springboard to teaching your child about people, behavior, values, right and wrong, and family expectations or standards. Again, you need not wait for your child to ask a question. I know of parents who, when watching television with their child, freely comment on the situations, ask the child questions, and reinforce family values that they want to convey to the child. For example, they might point out that a cartoon action is not real or that if it were real, someone would be badly hurt. They might ask what was good about that person's behavior or what was bad or whether the child would like that person for a friend. The idea is to talk about the meaning of the images on the screen and use them to teach facts and family values. This suggestion does not imply that you should allow your children to watch television without restriction. It simply shows that, if you are ready and willing to engage your child, even child- and family-oriented programs and commercials provide many teachable moments.

Challenges

Television, news broadcasts, and public discussions involving sex can trigger unexpected and complicated sexual questions from very young children, leaving you confused and anxious. You may feel paralyzed because the topic seems too complex for your child's comprehension, for example, gay and lesbian issues, orgasm, abortion, AIDS, pornography, infidelity, and so on. Although we all might prefer to wait until our child is more mature to explain some of these issues, the so-called premature questions are likely to come up in today's society.

These topics may be upsetting because we think we do not know enough or are uncertain about our values. Preparation is the key, and that is why this book had you work through the first three chapters. From these you began to understand and resolve personal inhibitions or concerns as a way of preventing extreme emotional reactions to your child's sexual situations. You began to build a team effort involving both parents or caregivers, if available, in order to work together on your child's sex education. You started the process of clarifying the sexual values and moral standards that you want to pass on to your child. All of these preparations, and the section you just read on the big sexual topics, give you a head start in finding the right words for your talks. The rest of this chapter teaches specific communication skills to help you translate your message into simple and brief responses that a young child can understand. And in the final section, you will have the opportunity to think about, rehearse, and become comfortable with the material.

The unique qualities of a child, his or her parents, the family structure, the physical environment, and the family's cultural, ethnic, or racial heritage may also give rise to specific learning needs and challenges. Depending on these, you should tailor your child's sex education accordingly. For example, a child who, from a young age, has a consistently "headstrong" or oppositional temperament may need much more structure, more careful parental supervision, and heavier doses of moral guidance than an easygoing, compliant child. Or a single parent who is dating may have to explain, even to a young child, what her dating means. If a parent, relative, or close family friend is gay or lesbian, a child may need a brief explanation about sexual orientation at an early age.

Another challenge that parents mention is the worry that their child will ask sexual questions in public places or will "blabber" to other kids, relatives, or neighbors the sexual information parents have taught. Both of these situations can be unsettling; however, the preparations you have done so far may have reduced such concerns. The unwelcome or untimely question (from your point of view) could come during church, in the supermarket, in a restaurant, at the zoo, or anywhere else, because young children don't censor their thoughts. Keep calm. Praise the question. ("That's a good question," or "I can see why you're asking that.") Answer briefly but accurately. Say that you will talk more about it when you get home or that you will read the book together again to get more details. The typical young child will not persist once you have offered some information and promised more.

One parent recently explained that she worried about teaching the correct names for genitals or explaining pregnancy or intercourse because she just knew her five-year-old son would run out and tell all this to his friends. In other words, she was embarrassed from just anticipating criticism from others. If this issue troubles you, ask yourself if the first three chapters in this book have helped you overcome the sense that accurate sexual information is somehow shameful, unseemly, or inappropriate for children to know. If you have begun to resolve some of these negative feelings, then you will likely find the right words to defend your choice to give sexual facts and guidance to your child.

One final challenge may arise if grandparents live in the family home or provide child care. You will need to make the older generation aware of the sex education you are offering and how you prefer to handle the child's sexual questions or situations. Be willing to have a dialogue about this emotional subject, explain your rationale, and engage in further conversations as necessary.

Parent Communication and Interaction Skills

Some parents might assume that high-level communication or relationship skills are not essential to being effective as a young child's sex educator. This view is probably correct in comparison to the demands of sustaining a meaningful conversation about sex with a teenager. Yet each stage of child development calls on you to respond in ways that match the child's intellectual abilities. This means that you have to be flexible and constantly adapt your communication to fit the child's cognitive and emotional level.

With the young child, the overarching and essential parental quality is the ability to provide good care, love, and nurturance. This is a tough job. It takes time, energy, patience, and emotional maturity. You have to put the child's needs first and be emotionally present, that is, tuned into the child, not spaced out in your own moods or preoccupations. This means your frustrations and dreams must often play second fiddle to the child's song of growing up.

Starting with your child's infancy, you provide good care that lays the foundation for your child to gain a healthy sexual life. Good care emerges with your every attention to and interaction with him or her: tenderly comforting or rocking your crying child; feeding, changing, bathing, and cuddling your little one; talking, singing, and playing games with your toddler; and answering the endless questions of your growing child. Most parents are able to offer this quality of child care, but not all. Abused and neglected children struggle to reach the milestones of physical and emotional development, and, for many, their sexual journey will be strewn with land mines.

In addition to promoting loving and compassionate child care, I have a few suggestions about communication skills that are directly relevant to your child's sex education. If you have begun to identify and resolve any personal sexual concerns that might cause embarrassment or anxiety and if you understand your child's need to know as part of normal development, then talking effectively about sex will come naturally after a bit of practice.

The single most important skill for parents is to assume the stance of teacher. Stated simply, your child's need to learn a few facts about sexuality is part of the need to learn about many things in the world. For example, the child who asks where babies come from does not have the adult perspective or emotions about sex, passion, intercourse, and all the complicated feelings that go with sexual experience. He or she just wants to understand how people get a baby. The following guidelines will help you enter and stay in the "teacher" mode when you talk to your child about sexual matters.

1. Give simple praise and approval for your child's questions about everything and for his or her listening, learning, and following rules. Do the same with sexual questions. This approach will encourage your child to bring any further sexual questions to you.

2. Expect the endless "why" questions about everything your child comes across or thinks about. This is normal behavior, and sexual questions are part of the need to name and understand how things work.

3. Explore, before answering, what your child's understanding is about the question. This lets you know what he or she is really asking and whether you need to correct a misunderstanding, add new factual details, emphasize your moral beliefs and standards, or do all of these.

4. Recall the attitude and tone that you use in teaching your child about such topics as foods, colors, numbers, words, family routines, cars, shopping, safety, and the like. Assume the same attitude and tone when you give basic sexual facts or answer sexual questions.

5. Be patient, use simple language, be brief, and get children's books that have the information along with pictures and drawings. That is, follow the same formula that works for teaching your child about other aspects of life.

6. When appropriate, briefly include your family's values, ideas of right and wrong, and rules for living, as you normally would with everything you teach, such as caring for pets, sharing toys, cleaning up, not littering, getting along with other children, showing respect for adults in authority, obeying laws, telling the truth, keeping a promise, and so on. Teaching your family's values and standards for all aspects of life lays the groundwork for the time when you will also teach about values as you answer sexual questions.

7. Expect to hear the same questions again, including sexual questions, and give them a welcome response. Repeated questions are normal. Your child's intellectual abilities and memory are still developing.

Practice Makes Perfect

Although most parents will likely see young children as the easiest age group to talk to about sex, practice is still necessary to build effective communication skills and get comfortable in sexual discussions. Several rehearsal exercises can prepare you before the curtain goes up on Act I of *My Life as My Child's Sex Educator*. Ideally, both parents or the parental team will use these exercises. The idea is not simply to read about them here but to actually carry them out as directed. So get a pad of paper and prepare yourself to write, get up and move around, telephone or meet with a friend, or talk with your partner or teammate.

Vocabulary Test

Determine the extent of your current usage of the correct names for the genitals by answering the following questions: What names do I use with my spouse or intimate partner? Have I ever used terms like *penis, scrotum, vulva,* or *vagina* in a discussion with a close friend, a physician, nurse, or other person? Do I flinch when I see these words in print?

List the occasions in which you have actually said aloud the names of men's and women's sexual and reproductive organs.

Mirror Talk

Look in a mirror and say aloud the aforementioned names for the genitals. For future use, add additional terms: clitoris (pronounced KLIH-ta-rus), hymen, cervix, urethra, uterus (womb), ovary, ovum (egg), fallopian tubes, menstruation, lubrication, orgasm, pubic hair, foreskin, testicles, semen, sperm, erection, and ejaculation. Do this exercise several times, and pay attention to your reaction.

Duets

. Talk to a close friend, spouse, or intimate partner about using these terms. Explain your initial emotions in response to saying the words in the Mirror Talk exercise. Ask about the other person's reaction and if, when, and where he or she uses these terms.

Make up some ordinary (or not so ordinary) conversations in which you might use the words with someone. Try the following suggestions, then make up your own, and feel free to laugh in the process. "I've been having an itching sensation in my vagina." "Honey, will you teach Andy to wash his penis and show him how to pull back the foreskin?" After practicing, you and your friend or partner can then discuss when or in what situations you would use some of these terms with your child.

Main Attractions

Consider all the major sexual topics we've discussed in this chapter that you will likely talk about with your youngster: naming and explaining the sexual organs, touching, toilet training, masturbation, nudity, body safety, playing doctor, where babies come from, and obscene words. For each topic, rate your current ability to discuss it with your young child (or imagined child) and your comfort level. Use this rating scale: 1 = can handle; 2 = worry about this one; 3 = wish to avoid; 4 = unprepared and unwilling. The ratings should suggest how much further preparation you need to do.

"Gag" Lines

Imagine the worst question your young child could ask or the worst scenario for one of the topics that you rated as 1 ("can handle") in the previous exercise. Practice aloud your child's and your own responses. Next, imagine your child asking about your personal sexual history or sexual life in regard to the same topic or another that you think you can manage. Remember both your right to privacy and your personal boundaries and your child's need to know a few basic sexual facts. Practice aloud your child's and your own responses.

More "Gag" Lines

Imagine additional sexual topics that your child might "prematurely" ask because of exposure to television, news reports, or public discussions of sexual matters (for example, gay and lesbian issues, orgasm, abortion, AIDS, criminal sex offenses, pornography, infidelity, oral sex, or anal sex)—for example, "Mommy, what is gay?" First, think through your factual understanding of sexual orientation. Decide whether you need more information. Then think through all aspects of your value position on this issue. Decide if you are clear on the value or ethical position that you want to pass on to your child. Using adult language, speak out loud with a message that reflects your understanding and values. Then speak out loud again, this time translating the message into a simple, brief answer to the child's question. Practice several times. Then move on to another "tough" topic.

More Duets

Consider all the major topics in the Duets exercise and ask your spouse, intimate partner, parental teammate, or a close friend (or organize a mothers' discussion group) to role-play with you question-and-answer scenes in which you and your child talk about the various topics. Start your role play by imagining the setting, the time, who's present, and what triggers the question or discussion—for example, something on television, a family situation, your child's behavior, or a question out of the blue. Then take turns with both of you having a chance to play the part of child and parent. Consider the "tough" unexpected topics and practice role plays with these too.

The Moral of the Story

Go back to each of the practice exercises and ask yourself two questions: Did I convey a simple but accurate explanation of the sexual topic? Did I also include, in an effective way that my child could understand, a moral or ethical viewpoint about this aspect of sexuality and any rules or standards of conduct that I want my child to learn? If you did not do both, practice the scenes again until you have conveyed the full message that you want your child to have. For example, in an explanation of where babies come from, after a simple explanation of the facts, a moral position might be "A husband and wife decide to make a baby only when they are grown-up adults and know they can take care of the baby and give it a good life." In other words, you might want to include a simple rule that reflects your values about love, commitment, marriage, intercourse, and having a baby. Obviously, you will find many more opportunities to convey your sexual values and moral code throughout your child's development, but you can start this process early on.

From this chapter's discussion of early childhood development, the importance of good parenting, your role in explaining the big sexual topics, teachable moments and opportunities, effective communication skills, and practice exercises, you should feel better prepared to help your child get a head start toward a healthy and morally sound sexual life.

Sex education at this stage is embedded within all aspects of child care. It is not just a talk or even a series of talks about sex. The first duty of parents and caregivers is to provide the loving, compassionate nurturance that builds the foundation for the child's sexual development. The child who attains a childhood conscience, a positive sense of gender identity, and an understanding of a few basic sexual facts can move smoothly into middle childhood and continue the journey to sexual health.

5

Teaching Kids from Six to Eleven

Tommy and Terry sitting in a tree,
K-i-s-s-i-n-g.
First comes love,
Then comes marriage,
Then comes Terry with a baby carriage.

If you watch TV, they've got everything you want to
know. . . . That's how I learned to kiss, when I was
eight. And the girl told me, 'Oh, you sure know how
to do it.'"
    Brett (age fourteen), quoted in Time, June 15, 1998

Middle childhood offers a bit of a breather with regard to the emotional energy demanded of parents. During the ages of about six to eleven, kids don't need the intense personal care required in the previous stage, and the turmoil of puberty and adolescence has not yet arrived to challenge parental confidence. Perhaps because your children spend all day in school, and the evenings busily pass with homework, activities, and family routines, you may not sense any urgency to provide sexual information. But even the busiest youngsters are continuing to develop into sexual beings. Recall your experiences during this stage of life:

- How did you learn about intercourse?

- Did you learn about menstruation during elementary school or before you got your first period?

- Did you see any pornography during your elementary or middle school years?

- What age were you when you and your friends started talked about pregnancy and childbirth?

- What age were you when you or your friends started to pay attention to the opposite sex?

- Do you remember your earliest, perhaps vague, romantic feelings, sensations, and fantasies?

- Did you have crushes on boys, girls, men, women?

Even without the pervasive sexuality that dominates today's culture, by age nine or ten you were probably curious about sex, learning in bits and pieces; by age eleven, you were likely taking a second look at certain people. You can be sure that youngsters in this age group are aware of the sexual aspects of life.

Middle childhood is the ideal time to prepare youngsters for the powerful winds of change and rising emotional tides that will come with puberty. It might be tempting to enjoy the calm as long as your child makes no sexual waves, but this is not a good idea. Although a few social critics think that children at this stage don't need sexual information and that puberty requires only the most basic sexual information,[1] I strongly disagree with this view.

Waiting for the first signs of maturing or the right time to have "the talk" is to waste valuable years and opportunities for guiding children about sex and morality. Without ongoing brief comments or sexual talks with parents, twelve-year-olds may not feel comfortable asking sexual questions even though they desperately need answers. One expert believes that by age six, children often surmise that they get no straight answers from parents and thus learn to keep silent about sexual activities or feelings.[2]

By reading this book, you are making sure that this doesn't happen to your child. This chapter enables you to continue the good work of being your child's sex educator and moral guide. You will gain

- Understanding of the emotional needs of kids living in the "neutral zone"

- Additional sexual information for carrying out your role in teaching about sex and morality for this age level

- Awareness of the unique teachable moments, opportunities, and challenges

- Additional communication and interaction skills to capitalize on kids' desire to learn

- Practice opportunities for improving and perfecting these skills

Children in the "Neutral Zone": Needs and Characteristics

When a child is six to eleven years old, his or her major emotional task is to gain a sense of competence through learning. Erik Erikson, the child development theorist whom I mentioned in Chapter Four, sees the challenge as a crisis in which children either achieve a sense of *industry* (which promotes competence) or are left with a sense of *inferiority*.[3] Their job is to learn about and master the facts of their world. Without the basic tools that come from learning, they will lack the ability to live successfully in their environment, and their overall emotional health will suffer.

The facts of human sexuality are part of the environment and part of school subjects, such as science, which includes human biology and health, and social studies, which includes the study of family groups that socialize children. And of course reading, which includes literature, explores love and other sexual themes.

Middle childhood is in a sense a neutral zone in terms of the sexual atmosphere surrounding the child and the parent-child relationship. During this relatively calm period, most children can take in large amounts of sexual information and accept moral guidelines without embarrassment or strong emotional responses. You should capitalize on the fact that children in this stage can be as neutrally curious about human sexual growth and development as they are about science, computers, weather, history, math, geography, and other subjects. If you have maintained a nurturing relationship, appropriate discipline, and moral authority, your child will readily respond to continued teaching about sexual facts and family standards of right and wrong.

How can you take advantage of the neutral zone to keep children on the road to a healthy and morally sound sexual life? First, you need to make sure your child gains competence, masters the learning that school and the family make possible, and reaps the immediate benefits that come with achievements. Second, you need to give big doses of information and moral guidance on a few sexual topics that children need to know about during this stage.

These two tasks suggest a natural partnership between parents and schools. Obviously, schools look to parents to help children stay focused on learning. Parents, in turn, should know how sexuality fits into the school curriculum, help develop and support sex education programs, and talk with their child about what he or she is learning about sex.

This point became meaningful to Jenna, a single parent who was visiting her son's third-grade classroom to help with a party. As several of the children came up to tell her they were studying about the human body, one boy popped up, "But we aren't going to learn about sex or reproduction." Another child said, "But we did learn what the anus is." Jenna later discovered that according to the curriculum plan, the study unit should have introduced concepts related to reproduction and pregnancy.

Promoting Competence

Parents want their child to have a successful life, and know that a good education is essential to reaching that goal, but they may not know exactly how a child's sense of mastery can also improve chances for a happy and healthy sexual life. The child who learns and achieves in school develops a sense of competence, worth, and value. Because this confidence lets her see that she has a positive future and a place in the world, she keeps learning and forming future goals.

Part of understanding the environment includes understanding human relationships, having the ability to get along with people, and adhering to society's rules. Without social competence, a child will have difficulty putting knowledge and skills into practice, such as in a job or career that brings rewards. Jerome and Joanna are two children who struggled in different ways with competence.

Jerome began to dislike school, gave up on learning, and failed the fifth grade. During the summer, he started hanging out with older kids on the street and thought about getting into their gang. He enjoyed all the talk about drugs, fighting other gangs, and sex. He felt accepted and important to the friends he met on the street. In autumn he complained to his parents about going into the special remedial school program and began to skip school and lie about his activities.

Johanna didn't have any trouble learning school subjects. She could get B's and C's with little effort and often waited until the last minute to do schoolwork. In this way she got to spend more time with her friends. She argued with her parents about chores and rules, and even in the fourth and fifth grade tried to live according to what she could get by with. By sixth grade, she and her girlfriends were regularly planning slumber parties as an excuse for being away from home so they could meet older boys. As Johanna became more focused on the excitement of feeling "grown up," she began to see school as a waste of time.

What causes children like Jerome and Johanna to get derailed from achieving the academic and personal competence needed for a successful school and family life? Each child's situation is different, but the following are some of the factors:

- A chaotic family life or living environment (or both) that cannot nurture the child at any stage of life

- Lack of parental attention and involvement in the child's needs and life

- Lack of appropriate parental support, supervision, and discipline related to the child's schoolwork, chores, and social activities and friends

- Lack of attention by the school and parents to building the child's character and positive sense of self and identity

- Personality, temperament, or special health conditions of the child that make learning difficult, including learning self-management and conforming to social rules

- Lack of effective parental and school response to the child's unique characteristics that create risks to healthy development

As parents, we have a primary role in keeping our child moving in a wholesome direction in life. In regard to physical health, we automatically schedule routine medical checkups and immunizations against diseases. We need to think about healthy emotional and sexual development in exactly the same way. Children need certain "immunizations" to promote sexual health and moral soundness. And parents, not doctors or teachers, have the major responsibility for these.

Action Steps to Promote Competence

Dr. Mom and Dr. Dad need to administer the first vaccination, which is the formula that promotes competence and prevents inferiority. It strengthens the total child, which includes body, mind, and spirit. It counteracts the toxins of ignorance and lack of interest in learning, which can produce such damaging diseases as hopelessness and alienation. Everything that you do to help your child learn, master facts, and gain competence also supports healthy sexual development. Here are a few simple guidelines for parents that will help the vaccine "take."

1. Be a part of your child's school life. Know his or her subjects or classes and become well acquainted with your child's teachers. Attend school programs and parent-teacher conferences; if possible, volunteer to help with school needs.

2. Set clear and regular times and locations (not in front of the TV) for schoolwork and enforce them.

3. Help your child get organized to do schoolwork through support for good study habits (reminders to bring homework and necessary materials, and so on).

4. Help with homework only in minor ways (to be sure directions are clear, for example). For ongoing difficulties in completing schoolwork, meet with your child's teachers to develop a plan to help.

5. Encourage reading by reading to and with your child, visiting the library, and obtaining educational videos as well as entertaining ones.

6. Put meaningful limits on anything that could interfere with your child's learning. This means restricting television, computer and video games, excessive involvement with friends, excessive family responsibilities, or overinvolvement in organized youth sports or activities.

7. Encourage, support, and praise your child's good work and efforts. Do not nag, berate, or criticize.

8. Respect your child's unique interests, abilities, and limitations.

Your role in helping your child achieve the task of competence is critical to sexual development, not merely icing on the cake. Competence allows your child to listen to and make use of sexual information and your moral guidance. These should come from you in many forms, not simply "the talk" or even many talks. Although discussions are central, as the next section shows, they can be effective only when you come across as a caring, supportive, knowledgeable parent with moral authority and the wherewithal to set and enforce family standards.

The Role of Parents in
Teaching About Sex and Morality

As you recall the initial quotations in this chapter—the innocent childhood rhyme about sex set against the eight-year-old's boast of learning the technique of kissing from television—what are you thinking and feeling? That the world is sex-crazy? Sadness at the loss of childhood innocence, anger that your child will grow up too fast in this world, worry about your child's sexual future? Once you get past any initial troubling emotions, stay focused on solutions.

You can control a certain amount of your child's exposure to our sexualized culture, especially within your own home. Even if you restrict television, videos, movies, and the Internet, however, kids will still hear a lot about sex—from other kids, from commercials, from innuendoes in "family-oriented" entertainment, and from news and public discussion. Most of this exposure will not provide full or accurate sexual information. Instead, children pick up bits and pieces of information and numerous sexual myths and fantasies that go unchallenged. This is why we must make a point to truly *educate* them with sexual facts!

Because we now live in a different age, longing for the "good old days" is a waste of energy. The millennium clearly holds new risks to sexual health, and these go beyond the deadly HIV virus and AIDS and other serious STDs. The social and cultural atmosphere also carries contagions that can harm the psychological, emotional, and spiritual dimensions of the child's developing sense of self and identity, which are central to making moral decisions.

We cannot wait until adolescence to teach children about the meaning of love and commitment; about the personal maturity and resources it takes to have and raise a child; about the work, energy, and rewards that come with marriage or an intimate committed relationship; and about the need for good sexual decisions to help a person have a happy life. Without parental guidance, youngsters by the age of ten will already be mimicking pop culture's teachings about love, relationships, and life. Knowing what's out there in today's world, we must opt for the preventive track and prepare our sons and daughters to resist the risks to sexual health that come from early sexual intercourse, sexual myths, and media exploitation. This you do by administering the second immunization: a dose of accurate sexual information along with moral values and guidance.

At any stage of your child's development, you have two methods (not equally effective) for helping your child understand sexuality. First, you may wait for the child's questions about sex or for naturally occurring situations that imply the need for sexual discussion. In other words, you may do a lot of waiting and watching (and perhaps worrying). In the second and much better approach, you take charge, plan, and implement the kind of sex education you want your child to receive. This proactive method lets you inoculate your child before the risky toxins and contagions can take hold and attack healthy emotional and sexual development.

The Booster Shot for Ages Six to Eight: Expanding on the Basic Facts

From about age six to eight, children begin to master facts about the world in general, and parents should make sure that this learning spurt includes a few more details about sexuality and sexual morality. Two guidelines may be helpful. First, obtain new children's books, suitable for this age group, that deal with sexual facts. Your child will naturally welcome a new book about sex for "big" kids, especially one with diagrams and illustrations that make learning easy. Reading to and with your child lets you convey the sexual information and your moral views before your child possibly studies some of these concepts in school or church. Second, find out about the sex education curriculum for this level in your child's school so that you can relate this to your teaching, and make it a point to support the school's program.

For this age group, the sexual facts should expand the child's knowledge about such important topics as the human body and development, pregnancy and childbirth, sexual behavior, health risks, personal safety and skills, and sexual orientation. The discussion of these topics in the next sections is not comprehensive. Instead it aims to help you with several of the more difficult sexual topics and those that school programs may not cover.

The Body, Sexual Organs, and Development

For several reasons, children should learn the correct terms for the rest of the external genitals and some of the internal sexual organs. These are important for the new facts they will need about inter-

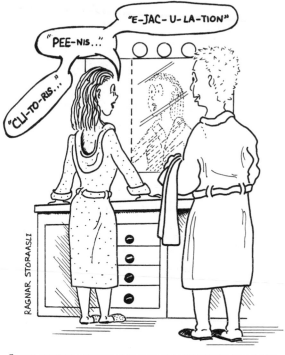

"I SEE YOU'RE REHEARSING FOR TONIGHT'S BIG SEX TALK
WITH THE KIDS."

course and pregnancy and for the later preteen information about puberty. Be prepared to use and explain *vagina, clitoris, uterus, ovary, ovum, semen, sperm,* and *erection*. Books with diagrams are essential. These will help your child learn that sexual organs have complicated internal parts and functions, just like other body organs, such as the parts that make hearing and seeing possible, the bones and muscles that support the whole body, and so on.

This is also a good time for reminders about the differences in boys' and girls' genitals and the importance and value of each gender. New teaching should include these concepts: bodies come in different sizes and shapes, kids grow at different rates, the body needs good nourishment to function and develop (air, water, food, exercise, and so on), and children should be proud of all that their body does. Such facts help young people develop a positive body image and learn healthy ways to make improvements. Parents need to give this message early and often. Weight and body image become a major concern for young people at puberty, especially for girls, who often start smoking and dieting in order to control weight.

When parents teach about sex in the context of understanding the whole body, they are also teaching moral lessons. Here are some ideas of right and wrong that your teaching conveys and that you may wish to emphasize:

- Information and knowledge are good.

- It is right to talk about sexual facts.

- It is good to go to books and materials for explanations of sexual matters.

- It is right to use correct terms and also to recognize that many other words exist for sexual organs and activity.

- Parents are a good source of sexual information.

- The body is a wonderful machine that is much more than its outward appearance.

- It's right to appreciate one's body and take good care of it through proper diet, exercise, and learning.

Pregnancy and Childbirth

Most parents are willing to teach their child at all ages about pregnancy and childbirth. Six- to eight-year-old children obviously need a few more facts beyond those given earlier, which I won't repeat here. But they should also begin to understand the more complex personal sexual behaviors and decisions that pregnancy brings. Often parents and school programs don't mention these or introduce them early enough to make a difference. Yet kids hear sexual words or ideas in everyday life that leave them wondering: "having sex," "knocked up," "the Pill," "test-tube baby," "abortion," and so on.

To make the information about pregnancy and childbirth meaningful, you should also touch on some of the more difficult areas, such as the choice to become pregnant and the responsibilities of having a child. With this proactive approach, mothers and fathers, rather than other kids or television, take control of explanations and lay the foundation for their child's further learning.

Thus children in the six- to eight-year-old range need to know that *sexual intercourse* is the means by which sperm, carried by semen, get to the egg to fertilize and start a baby. You also need to include other, more personal information:

- Every act of intercourse has the potential to cause pregnancy.

- Pregnant mothers need good health care.

- The typical birth takes place through the vagina, though sometimes through Cesarean birth.

- It is possible to prevent pregnancy.

- Most adults choose how many children to have.

- Choosing to get pregnant is a very important decision.

- Raising a child is a demanding, lifelong task.

- A woman who is unable to raise a child may give it up for adoption or end the pregnancy through abortion.

Because you will likely want to start early to give your moral values regarding pregnancy, your child needs this basic sexual information in order to make sense of your values and moral standards. From this factual framework, you can move on to giving your moral perspective and rules about sexual intercourse and pregnancy.

Remember that children this age like facts and find them fascinating, but they also need and respond to simple and clear rules of conduct. For example, they need to know the *fact* that unmarried or young people sometimes do have intercourse and that this can cause unwanted pregnancy. At the same time, with regard to *moral standards* about sexual intercourse that you believe in for your child, he or she needs to hear these stated in clear and simple language.

Unless you totally oppose marriage on philosophical grounds, this is not the time to go into detailed distinctions between marriage and committed relationships of various kinds. At this stage, many parents who intend to make such distinctions later with older teenagers will use the term *marriage* as a shorthand term that young children understand to explain their belief that sexual intercourse is for adults who will stand by each other. For example, I know of parents, including those who are single or divorced, who teach the following moral lessons: that sexual intercourse is part of marriage (add a religious view if you wish); marriage is an important lifelong commitment; only adults are ready to make this commitment; and married adults are in the best position to choose whether to become pregnant and raise a child.

Because abortion is so much in the news, you should give a brief explanation and also give your specific moral view of the right course for an unwanted pregnancy. Obviously, other special characteristics of your child or family might lead you to present both the facts and your moral teachings about the topics of pregnancy and childbirth somewhat differently.

Sexual Behavior

Talking about sexual behavior has always been difficult for parents, primarily since it encompasses masturbation, "petting" or "making out," sexual intercourse, and the whole idea of genital pleasure. Because school sex education programs often cannot teach about these topics, parents have a responsibility to acknowledge the simple but often embarrassing fact that sexual behavior involves pleasure. Without this concept, they may not be able to explain other aspects of sex or respond effectively to the child's sexual questions or situations.

Some children's books may introduce the idea of pleasure in sexual behavior in ways that are acceptable to parents and make their job easier. For example, in *Where Did I Come From?* Peter Mayle touches on this delicate subject by explaining that "making love" brings "a very nice feeling for both the man and woman" and goes on to describe "a gentle tingly sort of tickle," which ends "in a tremendous big lovely shiver for both of them."[4] If you are anxious about these words, you might ask yourself whether you prefer this type of explanation that presents a respectful account of how and why the sexual organs feel good when touched, or the alternative of teaching nothing, in which case your child learns whatever is circulating on the playground, on *Beavis and Butthead*, or in the many sexual scenes and innuendoes on television.

Acknowledging that sexual touch brings pleasure is also important because masturbation can be an issue during this stage. Some children may, on occasion, openly masturbate if they have not completely learned the earlier message about privacy or how to act on that knowledge. You will need to explain this again. Acknowledging the pleasure of sexual touch with kids in the neutral zone may clear the way for more thoughtful future talks with teens, who watch closely for signs of parental honesty and hypocrisy.

Serious Physical Risks to Sexual Health

The most serious risks to sexual health come from diseases that threaten life itself, HIV and AIDS, and from other STDs that can have damaging effects on the sexual and reproductive systems. Teaching even young children about these diseases is part of the preventive immunization that parents must administer through sexual information and moral guidance. These topics are tough because infection takes place primarily through sexual behaviors that parents find difficult to talk about.

Thirty-four states mandate HIV-AIDS education in public schools, but one-half of these do not also mandate general sexuality education.[5] This means that parents in these seventeen states have to provide all the rest of the sex education that a child needs to understand how these diseases fit in the broader context of human sexuality. Moreover, even the mandated HIV-AIDS education programs may not begin until junior or senior high school.

For these reasons, and because the child will likely hear references to AIDS-HIV and other STDs, parents should plan to provide a few basic sexual facts about these diseases early on. Remember, your child is learning about other types of diseases and so has some framework for understanding. Briefly explain that these diseases, like others, result from infectious viruses and bacteria, that they are spread during certain kinds of sexual activity with an infected person, that the diseases can be prevented by not engaging in the risky sexual behaviors with an infected person, and that kids will need to know about this serious problem for their future adult life.

With these simple facts, you can then add your moral perspective, for example, by repeating that this risk is not a problem when sexual intercourse is kept within marriage or is between adults who are mature enough to deal with these grown-up matters. Again, facts and moral guidance should be simple, clear-cut, and not frightening to the child. Only you can decide whether unique conditions, such as having a close friend or relative with HIV-AIDS, demand more or less information than that suggested here.

Personal Body Safety

Body safety takes on new importance for the six- to eight-year-old child, yet we may hesitate to talk about this topic. Since it elicits our own worry about our child's safety and well-being, we wonder if discussion about it will make our child anxious about daily life or fear sex in adult life. We can overcome this worry somewhat by providing a comprehensive account of sexuality, as this lets children understand body safety in a balanced way.

During this life stage, children begin to spend more time away from home—in school, in after-school activities, in visits with friends and relatives, or at home alone with baby-sitters or siblings. You need to update and expand the earlier information, continuing to explain that the child owns his own body and that no older kid or adult, except parents or medical persons (for good reason), can look at or touch his private parts. Reminders are in order, as well as more details that help the child protect himself. You should explain the following:

- How an adult might use children's interests or games to try to entice them into sexual activity

- How to leave immediately if inappropriate touch happens and not worry about hurting the person's feelings

- How to tell someone else about a touch that doesn't feel right

- Why secrets don't apply to this kind of situation

- That it is never a child's fault if this happens

Older siblings who look after a child should know this same information and more. They need to understand their responsibility to provide good care in the absence of parents.

Before age ten or twelve, many children will have heard about some child, perhaps even a close friend or relative, who experienced sexual abuse. Parents will need to talk openly, sensitively, and factually about such an occurrence and provide support for their child who may find this situation upsetting. (Chapter Three discussed the special needs of a child who has been sexually abused and how parents should tailor their sex education to address this unique characteristic.)

The moral lessons for the topic of body safety are obvious: the child owns his or her body, including private sexual parts; it is wrong for an older or stronger person to take advantage of a child; it is wrong for people to exploit others in sexual ways; it is right to protect yourself, stop the abuse, and tell; and child abuse, molestation, and rape are not just wrong—they are also crimes.

Another moral element for parents centers on how to convey the positive dimensions of sexuality while also giving this serious message. You don't want to frighten your child or come across as connecting sexuality simply to danger or evil. As mentioned before, the positive, normal, and enriching dimensions of sexuality come through when you start early to treat sexuality as a routine part of the child's learning and when you explain its many aspects. This comprehensive sex education will balance the realistic risks and dangers.

Sexual Orientation

Do you think your child has heard the words *lesbian, gay, homosexual*; seen news reports of gay pride groups; and heard reference to violence or "hate crimes" against gay men? Sexual orientation has triggered much controversy in public and political discussions. Some people think that schools should not teach anything about homosexual or bisexual orientations, especially at the elementary school level. Parents who recognize that children hear and wonder about this topic should prepare by obtaining facts and clarifying their moral position well ahead of time. As suggested in previous chapters, the gay, lesbian, and bisexual orientations have existed in all cultures, along with the predominant heterosexual orientation. And sexual orientation presumably results from multiple interacting factors during fetal or early childhood development to influence which sexual orientation a person will have.

Simply put, the child needs parents to acknowledge, not deny or avoid, the *facts of sexual orientation:* most people are attracted romantically and sexually to the opposite sex, but others have these feelings for the same sex, or sometimes for both sexes. You can also explain that sexual orientation is one of several qualities that make people unique, such as physical characteristics; cultural, ethnic, or racial background; personality; and education level. You can also remind your child of the general moral-ethical principle that all human beings have value and are more alike than different. You may wish to go beyond this brief ethical and moral viewpoint or do so when your child is older.

The Preteen Vaccination: The Facts of Puberty and More

Between the ages of nine and eleven, children need preparation for the coming growth spurt that will bring intense focus on their bodies and feelings. Because the emotional turmoil that comes with puberty can cloud their factual knowledge, you as a parent should help them "cram" as many sexual facts as possible—while they are still able to relate to the information as "facts." Thus a girl who has a complete and positive understanding of the details of menstruation is more likely to adapt quickly to the reality of monthly periods, rather than experience this change as an assault on her body integrity.

Stated figuratively, look at your nine-year-old as a pier that you're constructing on the beach. You need to build the foundation with reliable and durable materials, because the high tides of adolescence can erode even the strongest foundation. Tap other resources to help with this task. Schools, health and wellness programs, and community youth agencies often provide educational programs designed specifically to help parents and children prepare for puberty. Once again, the discussion that follows is not comprehensive. Instead, it focuses on a few sexual topics that parents rarely touch, including values that can affect the long-range sexual happiness of young people.

More Information and New Information

With preteens, the major ingredient in the vaccination formula consists of detailed information about the changes to expect at puberty, specifically, physical appearance; menstruation; wet dreams;

and a variety of feelings about one's body, sexual sensations, and attraction and interest in others. It should also include further facts about the human body and sexual organs; reproduction, pregnancy, childbirth, and birth control; the consequences of teen pregnancy; sexual behavior; health risks from STDs; personal safety and skills to protect themselves; and sexual orientation.

The best way to make sure that your child gets all this information is to obtain and read with your child a comprehensive sex education book geared to preteens. ("Sex Education Resources" in the Resources suggests several titles, for example *Dr. Ruth Talks to Kids: Where You Came From, How Your Body Changes, and What Sex Is All About.*) Remember, your child is eager to learn about everything at this stage. And a book covers the facts, leaving you in a good position to discuss not only the facts but also your family's moral values and expectations. Because I think a good book is the parent's best resource for covering the details of puberty, I do not cover these explanations here, but will focus more how you can foster healthy emotional development.

Even when your child is at puberty, you wonder how much information to give him or her. Sometimes your child will let you know. Lisa was feeling good about having explained the facts of menstruation during the past year to her eleven-year-old daughter, Lauren. They had talked about body changes and sanitary protection, and Lauren had been very receptive to the information. Then, several months later, Lauren raised some questions as her mom was driving her home from school.

LAUREN: Does it hurt to take a tampon out?

LISA: No, not really.

LAUREN: Well, does it hurt to put it in?

LISA: No, you learn how to do this, and with practice, it doesn't hurt.

LAUREN: Then it doesn't hurt when a penis goes in either?

LISA: (stammering) Well, uh. I don't think I can answer that right now and drive safely at the same time.

Lisa regretted that she hadn't gotten that far yet in her daughter's sex education, but she was glad she gave an honest answer about not being able to talk about it at that moment. This situation is a good argument for using a children's book that covers many aspects of sexuality. For example, a simple explanation from *Dr. Ruth Talks to Kids* could have answered Lauren's question at the same time she was learning about puberty: "Because the vagina creates its own moisture when a woman is sexually aroused, the penis goes in easily."[6]

Information and Personal Meaning

Besides gaining new information, preadolescents need to hear about the personal and emotional meanings that we assign to sex, specifically what it tells us about ourselves and about how it fits with interpersonal relationships. Youngsters in middle childhood are beginning to gain a sense about how sexual feelings make them feel toward themselves and others. Parents rarely talk in depth about these personal meanings, although these will obviously affect the long-range sexual happiness of young people. (Some highly personal meanings about sex appeared in Chapter Two, which advised fathers to help their sons maintain a positive self-image as they contend with worries about the penis and secondary sexual characteristics, masturbation and wet dreams, fantasies, and managing intense emotions.)

The following discussion highlights topics that bear directly on the child's understanding of how sex affects self and relationships and the moral and ethical implications of these. Teens themselves say they wish parents would talk to them about boy-girl relationships, specifically about emotions and commitment. So beyond all the basics, when you can talk about what sex means to human beings and their relationships, you are laying a foundation for more complex talks about this subject with teenagers. Now is the time to give your ideas about the deep emotional and spiritual meanings of sexuality that go beyond what the popular culture portrays. Remember that with preteens, such remarks may arise as passing comments and don't have to produce detailed discussions or debates. Instead, you can offer a piece of information, talk and respond to questions, and then briefly and simply give your moral view and make clear your expectations for your child.

In covering the following topics, I speak directly to young people and separately tailor the messages for boys and girls. The content draws on research and ethical values based on behavioral science's approach to sexual health (which you briefly considered in Chapter Three).

This format, which includes both information and values, can serve as an example of how you might phrase these and other ideas. They could be part of a discussion about nearly any sexual topic. *Do not think of these as parental speeches or lectures,* but simply as ideas that you might include in bits and pieces in give-and-take discussions. In such a dialogue, you would also be asking for and listening to your child's views or experiences with these sexual matters. Naturally, you could also choose to further link the ethical message more specifically to religious beliefs that you endorse.

Messages with Meaning for Preteen Boys

Early on, you can help your son understand a few facts and moral and ethical guidelines about his sexuality, the nature of intimate relationships, and personal responsibility. Consider these three examples and think of other messages along these lines that you want to give.

Sex Is Serious Business Puberty means that you begin to have the appearance of an adult while you're still trying to grow up and learn the ropes about the world, and this fact can cause problems for kids. This means that standards have changed for how you can behave. You have to pay close attention to your feelings, the way you conduct yourself with boys, girls, children, and adults in private and in public. Growing up means that you are responsible for the way you behave and your decisions. This means you need to think about a behavior and the possible results. If you behave in a sexual way with another person, it can be a serious matter.

Sometimes boys use sexually suggestive, obscene, or threatening language; or sexually approach, touch, or grab another person without her consent; or even mimic sexual activity as humor, joking, and so on. You may see this stuff in the media, but it doesn't fly in real life. All of these behaviors could result in charges of sexual harassment or even criminal charges. So regardless of whether you think such a behavior is a joke or horseplay with a group of friends, you need to realize that you have a choice about how you behave. In our family, we expect you to respect yourself and others and know that sexual behavior of that kind is not a joking matter. Sex is private and takes place between people who care about and love each other and give their consent.

Treat Girls as People Growing up means you will likely take an interest in girls, want to get to know them, want them to like you, and feel sexually attracted to them. These are all normal feelings. As you are still trying to learn about yourself, make a point to learn about and appreciate girls as people, not as simply female bodies to look at and fantasize about. Although you might hear other boys (and girls) talk about girls' bodies; criticize, label with slurs, and joke about them; leer at or make obscene gestures toward them; and boast about having sex with them, I expect you to treat girls as you would any friend whom you care about and as you want to be treated. You can learn a lot about girls, about how they think, and about life by making friends with them. In our family, we expect you to treat all people with respect.

You're Responsible Sex with another person carries great responsibility, for both you and your partner. This means you can get hurt and mess up your own and your partner's life if you don't make good decisions about sex. Sexual relationships are for mature adults who can handle the responsibility and any consequences. Young people are not ready for all of this.

Remember, deciding to engage in a sexual relationship means you accept 100 percent responsibility for yourself and your partner. You must count on yourself for protection from pregnancy and disease; for talking honestly about what the sex means; for your and your partner's feelings afterward about yourselves, each other, and the relationship; for any pregnancy or disease that might result; for others' finding out; and for any upsetting of life plans for either of you. That's a lot of responsibility, and sex is not a game or pastime. We believe you will have a happier life, including your sex life, by waiting until you are mature enough to take on all these responsibilities. In our family, we expect you not to engage in sex with a partner until you are an adult [or married].

All three of these messages suggest both information and moral guidelines that you might give to your son. As mentioned before, don't look on these thoughts as one-time lectures. These ideas should come up in numerous talks with your child. For example, here's a conversation a mother had with her ten-year-old son.

MOM: Your cousin John is going to be a father. You know his girlfriend is pregnant.

SON: Yeah, I heard Dad tell you.

MOM: I wish he had given more thought to what could happen to his and Lori's life when he decided to have sex at age sixteen.

SON: Well, it's not your problem.

MOM: Yes, but I'm sorry that they have such a big problem to deal with. It causes me to think about your future. You know what your dad and I think about this. Sex is for adults who are old enough to take care of themselves and be responsible for the consequences. I expect you to follow that belief in your own life as you get older. Give yourself time to grow up and learn how to make good decisions about sex. Waiting until you are mature enough will make your life better when you're a teenager and as an adult too.

SON: I'm outta here.

Messages with Meaning for Preteen Girls

If boys need to hear messages about responsibility and caring empathically for others, girls may very well need to hear messages about responsibility to themselves. You can begin, even with a preteen, to help her appreciate and nurture her unique identity and not deny or devalue her sexuality in return for a relationship. Consider these three messages, remember that you could fit them within discussions about various sexual topics, and think of other messages along these lines that you want to give.

Appreciate Your Body When you start to grow up, your body will change and become more feminine and have more body fat and curves. This is the way women's bodies are supposed to be. These are the physical qualities that make a healthy pregnancy possible. Take care of your body in healthy ways with exercise and good food. Don't buy into the commercial images of thin women as models of the only way to be attractive. These images appeal to emotions and fantasies in order to sell stuff to people who are stupid enough not to know they are being manipulated. Your body takes care of you; be proud of it and take care of it.

Tune In to Your Identity and Sexuality As you grow up, you will have many emotions, thoughts, fantasies, and sensations in your body, such as in your sexual organs. This is also the time when you will begin to learn a lot about yourself, discover your interests and talents, sort out your hopes and dreams for what you want to be or do as an adult, and work in school to reach those goals. Learning about your sexuality and sexual feelings is part of this too, such as through masturbation. Your sexuality belongs to you and is a normal part of your whole identity and personality. We want you to take time to get to know the true you that's inside and to become all that you want to be.

Treat Boys as Friends, Not Just Potential Boyfriends Sometimes as girls start to grow up, they obsess about having a boyfriend. It's normal and fun to like and fantasize about a particular boy or boys. You will probably like boys and find a lot of them attractive. This is a time when you and your friends may talk a lot about getting a boy to go with you, who likes who, and so on. The talk part can be fun, but getting paired up is not the only good outcome. Take time to learn about boys, become friends with different types of boys, see what qualities you like, watch how they treat people, and notice whether they share your interests and appreciate your abilities. You know we don't believe in young kids pairing up, starting to date, and spending a lot of time with one partner. That's why we will have rules about this.

Thus far you have seen how you can interact with kids who inhabit the neutral zone of middle childhood. You have reviewed some of the important sexual topics that you should cover with your six- to eight-year-old child. Then you considered ways to help preteens counter the powerful adolescent tendency to conform to rigid stereotyped sexual identities and superficial notions about relationships. These often influence their sexual decisions during adolescence and adulthood in ways that interfere with a healthy sexual life.

Sexual facts (as presented in books and your talks), along with discussions of your clear moral values and family rules, make up the vaccine for this stage of life. The question is exactly how to admin-

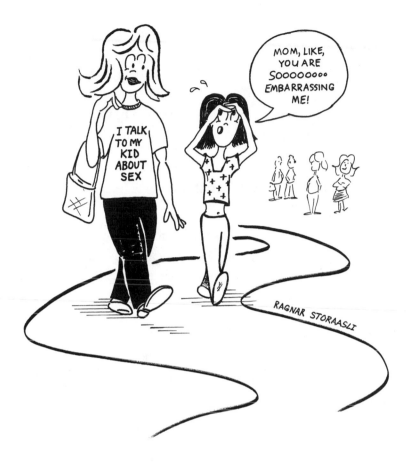

ister it. The next section will make you aware of the opportunities and challenges of the neutral zone; it includes further ideas and examples of other important sexual topics.

Teachable Moments, Opportunities, and Challenges

The reassuring thing about the neutral zone is that typically kids are receptive to learning and to adults' ideas. Because this attitude gives you an advantage that may not continue throughout adolescence, you should make the most of it. The qualities of youngsters in this stage suggest various ways to incorporate sexual information and moral guidelines. Children in elementary school love facts, new words, and concrete pictures or diagrams about how things work. They are open to new experiences, they like games, and they warm up to both competition and cooperation. They have a sense of humor, which, unfortunately, sometimes disappears for a while in adolescence.

Parents as Planners and Initiators

Although many teachable moments will arise, especially after your child has obtained some basic sexual information, you should also plan and initiate your child's sex education. Although I have already mentioned some of these, here is the full set of specific guidelines for this role.

1. Obtain sex education books geared for your child's age. Go the bookstore alone and review several books. Purchase at least one that you like, and then buy another geared to the next advanced level, for future use (or for backup if you have an inquisitive child). You can also obtain additional books from the library or educational videos, but a child should have at least one book for keeps.

2. Read the book with your child as part of the normal reading routine, perhaps at bedtime or instead of television. Keep the book out, along with others, that are favorites. You don't have to read it all at one time, and you can pick it up to read with the child more than once. Explore for what are the most fascinating facts, and add and talk about your moral views all along.

3. Suggest other children's literature that deals with feelings, growing up, and life. Children's novels by Judy Blume have long been favorites with kids, for example, *Are You There God? It's Me, Margaret.* Encourage your child to enter reading competitions at school or the library. Ask about your son or daughter's favorite books and what these stories have to do with life.

4. During meals or other family time, bring up a variety of interesting or controversial topics for discussion and use these to interact with your child and inform him or her. Then when you bring up sexual topics in the news, these will seem part of a normal family routine of talking about things. Look for opportunities to mention sexual topics, such as from something going on in the community, with friends or family, in the schools, in the news, or on television. Don't forget to explore reactions to sermons or studies at your place of religious worship.

5. Be active in discovering or creating other opportunities for discussions about sex, such as through your child's subjects of study or school projects. (Perhaps encourage a project on a topic such as the body, reproduction, child development, or parenting.) Take your child to museums or art galleries and talk about how early cultures approached family life, how art depicts the human body, and similar topics. Not all of this has to be about specific sexual lessons per se, but your child will see you talking rationally about many subjects and learn that you are an "askable" parent.

6. Learn about school, church, and community sex education programs for this age level. Review program goals and materials and, if you approve of them, enroll your child. Then follow up by talking with your child about what he or she is learning. You can also ask specifically from the teacher how parents can be involved.

Naturally Occurring Opportunities

Many opportunities for sexual discussion between parent and child arise in the course of family living and routines. Few teachable moments appear, however, if parents don't spend time with their children. Before considering examples of naturally occurring situations for teaching about sex, remember that the whole family atmosphere helps strengthen your child's moral conscience and ability for self-management. These qualities too are part of sexuality education.

Children in this stage need a home life in which parents have a strong presence and provide personal involvement, compassion, supervision, family rules, and protection. Simply explaining values and expectations for behavior can be just empty words if parents don't provide the necessary structure and supervision to enable children to live by the family's standards. This applies to how much time children are left alone, allowed to be with friends, and allowed to be in situations without parental supervision or that of other known and trusted adults. Good sex education and moral guidance demand parents who are present and know about and make decisions as to their child's permitted activities, schedule, and whereabouts.

Young people benefit from regular family routines for schoolwork, chores, bedtime, and leisure time. Their lives and sense of belonging are enriched by simple but meaningful family rituals surrounding birthdays, holidays, visiting relatives, going to church, and family picnics or other special events. When parents create a stable and wholesome family atmosphere, they readily find opportunities to help their child master sexual facts and live by the family's moral standards.

I recently heard about how a parent responded to her child's "naturally occurring" behavior to teach an important lesson.

> Krissa was becoming more and more annoyed about her eight-year-old daughter Kendra's constant talk about getting lipstick, nail polish, and "sexy" fashions. Krissa had calmly explained several times that these were not appropriate for Kendra's age, and Krissa herself didn't pay excessive attention to these aspects of feminine appearance. Still Kendra persisted in begging. When Kendra later explained that many of her girlfriends at school were starting to use makeup, Krissa then talked about peer pressure and television images of women and girls and repeated their family's values and behavioral standards. Finally, she also told Kendra the clear conse-

quences to expect if she continued to beg for these things.

Teachable moments can come up naturally, but you have to be present and tuned in to recognize them.

> Maureen was cooking dinner with her two children, Melissa, fifteen, and Mark, eleven, when Melissa complained about how guys will do or say almost anything to get girls to have sex with them. Maureen decided that Mark was the one who needed a message, so she said, "Mark, I want you to remember that this kind of behavior is wrong. When you're older and in a relationship, I expect you to be honest about what your intentions are. It's wrong to take advantage of a person to get what you want. You heard what your sister said about guys' lying, fooling themselves, making false promises. Some guys even force sex, and that's rape. If and when you do decide to have sex, I want you be honest and protect yourself and your partner." Maureen later admitted that her words sounded like a lecture, but she figured this didn't hurt Mark because he listened very closely.

As examples throughout this book show, opportunities to talk about sexuality arise in routine family situations: doing homework, chores, or shopping; driving kids to school or activities; watching television and videos; and so on. So much of television centers on sexual images and content that you could probably have a continuous discussion about its messages. Think seriously about how this content affects children's developing sexuality, and take steps to counteract the content you oppose. Let your child know your values about the meaning of sex, love, and commitment in comparison to the way that pop culture presents intimate relationships. Start by setting reasonable restrictions on television time and shows permitted. Comment on and discuss demeaning, degrading, or stereotyped depictions of sexuality when these come up, even in approved programs. Ask about and discuss the morality of a character's behavior, whether a scene reflects real love or real life, whether a character would make a good husband or wife, and so on.

Challenges

Every family is different, and certain characteristics call for you to tailor your child's sex education to address certain unique family situations. (Recall from Chapter Three that parents will need to incorporate special guidelines to meet the needs of an early maturing, gay, or disabled youth or of a child with difficult personality traits, a past history of sexual abuse, or gender identity confusion.)

You must be similarly sensitive to any family or group cultural traditions, values, and beliefs having to do with sexuality and decide whether you endorse or oppose these as part of your child's sexual learning. For example, the Hispanic culture in general emphasizes strict gender roles, discourages open discussion of sexual matters, values virginity for girls, but also accepts premarital sexual activity for boys as part of the "Latin lover" myth. Yet as acculturation takes place, many Hispanic parents question aspects of their culture's sexual legacy and wish to prepare their children to cope with the greater personal freedom that is available to youth in the larger U.S. culture.[7] Cultural and racial perceptions may also complicate the sex education efforts of some inner-city African American parents. If the family lives in an environment that, for example, accepts early initiation of sexual intercourse and gives positive attention to pregnant girls and young mothers, parents who wish to prevent these outcomes for their child have to carefully plan their child's sex education. From the time the child is very young, the parents' task is to inoculate the child to withstand the sexual pressures, risks, and dangers that come with the environment. Obviously, this is no small venture.[8]

One additional challenge relates to your personal qualities. You should monitor your own unconscious collaboration with the demeaning or commercial values that the media and culture assign to sexuality. For example, do you contribute to the premature sexualization of your child by overemphasizing physical appearance, features, dress, and the latest fashions or by allowing young children to wear adult-style clothing or model the behavior of entertainers or pop celebrities? Do you make comments about children being in love, having sweethearts, being popular? With young children, these influences can begin to define their sense of self and beliefs about sexuality. If you don't counteract superficial messages about sex with your own values, media influences will almost certainly mold your child's identity. Rather than simply criticizing, you need to explain how a richer and more realistic view of sexuality and sexual relationships can lead to a happier, more satisfying life. Remember that premature sexualization of children detracts from their primary developmental task of gaining competence through learning.

Parent Communication and Interaction Skills

Talking about sex with a child in the neutral zone calls for additional communication skills beyond those you learned to use with younger children. Beyond the basic role of teacher, you will now advance to another level. First, for the sexual facts, assume the stance of a "resource teacher" who can help a child master special units of study and locate needed learning materials. Second, to promote your child's emotional and moral development, be just what you are: the parent who nurtures, supports, inspires, and sets and enforces rules of conduct. Because I have already listed specific guidelines for helping a child achieve competency and for creating a wholesome family atmosphere that supports the developing conscience, the focus here is on a few skills to capture a child's attention and make learning fun. These will help you make sexual discussion a routine part of your child's learning and show you how to start and sustain effective talks about these personal matters.

1. Use open-ended questions to start and maintain conversations about *many topics*, not just sex. Ask about school, friends, homework, projects, interests, hobbies, sports, and books or magazines. If you can't have easy conversations about many topics, don't expect to start this process with sex.

2. Use open-ended questions as well with sexual topics. "Did you see, read, or hear about . . . ?" Then listen and keep asking questions to check your child's understanding of the sexual issue.

3. Use Socratic questions. These are questions framed to stimulate children to think through and arrive at information or ideas that they already know. This approach works well for sexual discussions because a correct or reasonable answer can come from the child, not a parent or teacher. For example, "What is the significance of having two hundred million to six hundred million sperm in each ejaculation?" This type of question helps children arrive at meaningful connections between various sexual facts and also make connections between facts and moral issues.

4. Start talks with sexual information (the facts) and end with moral or ethical values and expectations. This approach is important whether you, your child, or a situation bring about a sexual discussion. This skill may go against the typical parental impulse to rush immediately to a judgment, warning, or rule. Focus on the facts first, help your child think about them, and check his or her understanding of them. *Then* begin to talk about your moral or ethical perspective and present clear standards for your child.

5. Throw out sexual "factoids" (a term used by CNN)—brief but intriguing facts a child should find useful, with or without further discussion. "Did you know that the United States has the highest teen pregnancy and childbearing rate of all developed nations?" "Did you know that one in four sexually active teens will contract a sexually transmitted disease before graduating from high school?"

Include positive aspects of sexuality too: "Did you know that by age fifteen, most teens are happy with their new development and feel good about themselves?"

6. Create other kinds of guessing games out of sexual facts. "In any given year, how many teens in America have a sexually transmitted disease?" (Answer: 2.5 million.) Develop true-false questions as another way to present a sexual fact, engage your child, and pique interest in sexual information.

7. Offer parental "monologues" on selected sexual topics. These are most effective when your child is in a captive position, such as in the car. In a monologue you simply talk, without necessarily expecting a response, about some sexual information that you've seen, how it applies to people, how it fits with your moral values, and how it applies to your family. The monologue is a way to let your child know about you, what you know about sex, and what your values are. You might start by saying, "I've been thinking about . . . and sorting out what it means to me." Afterwards, and if you get groans and complaints, simply say (in a lighthearted tone or one that reflects your style), "I'm just doing my job as a parent. I want you to know what I believe. I don't want you ending up in ten years telling some therapist that your mom never talked to you or never gave you any sex education or rules for life."

8. Use the "two-plus-two finish" as a way to end your discussions about sex. Here's how it works. "Tell me two things you learned from our talk that let you know how sex is a good part of life (or a positive part of human beings or a gift from God). Now tell me two things that you learned from our talk that let you know how people have to be careful about sex so it doesn't cause them trouble in life." The two-plus-two finish also puts the onus on you to present a balanced view of sexuality.

9. Use the quick pep talk or pep response. This can be very brief and works best after listening empathically to worries or bad feelings. Here are some examples. Compliment your child on learning, or talking, or his or her decisions, and mention how these efforts

help healthy development. Reassure your child about growing up, about his or her unique qualities, about discovering and respecting personal abilities and strengths, and about the good future that lies ahead. Also part of this is accepting that your child doesn't need to be perfect—for example, "Everyone has flaws and shortcomings, and we all make mistakes. That's part of being human. You have plenty of good qualities to be proud of."

10. Stay sensitive to your child's reaction so that you can judge how much to say and when to wrap up your talk. Expect these interactions to be quite brief sometimes. If you end on a positive note and stay in a good humor, other opportunities will come up again.

Practice Makes Perfect

Chapter Four, which deals with young children, offers several specific guidelines on how to rehearse and get ready to perform well in the role of sex educator and moral guide for your child. Those basic practice exercises can apply as well to honing skills for the neutral zone of middle childhood. The difference is that the child is older, and the sexual information and guidance need to be more detailed. Remember the importance of practicing the vocabulary of sex, using the mirror for this, using sexual terms or concepts with other people before talking with your child, rating your comfort level with various topics, imagining the worst sexual question your child could ask and practicing responses, rehearsing in a role play with your partner other question-and-answer talks, and rehearsing the exact moral values you want to convey in a given question or situation.

Use these same exercises when preparing to talk about additional facts that will upgrade your child's sexual knowledge and introduce new material. The topics for age six to eight are the internal as well as external sexual organs of boys and girls; pregnancy and childbirth; sexual behavior, including intercourse and masturbation; health risks of sexually transmitted diseases; personal body safety and skills; and sexual orientation. The main information for preteens includes detailed explanations about all the changes that puberty brings for boys and girls: physical appearance, menstruation, wet dreams, and a variety of feelings about one's body, sexual sensations, and attraction to and interest in others. In other words, with these more advanced sexual topics, begin your practice, as before, by getting comfortable with the vocabulary, using the terms with other people, imagining the worst question your child could ask, and so on.

A few new practice exercises can also help you even further refine the skills needed for the neutral zone. All of these are designed to enhance your competence as your child's resource teacher and boost your confidence for being a moral guide. The goal of this training is to identify any barriers that make a given topic difficult and to help you overcome these. Remember, you can do more than simply read about these exercises. Try them out and get your partner involved with you.

Basic Research

From one of the books you get on sexuality, prepare a set of sexuality facts, perhaps one for each of the topics mentioned in the introduction to these exercises, and put them on index cards. Then figure out how you might use each fact with your child (as a factoid, in a question-and-answer game, as a true-false question, or something else). Without this concrete preparation, you will never have a relevant fact handy or on the tip of your tongue when you most need one.

Overcoming Study Blocks

Think aloud, either privately or in the presence of a trusted spouse, partner, or close friend, about one of the main topics that is most troubling (one for which you rated yourself unprepared and unwilling to discuss). Speak about this sexual topic, as if in a stream of consciousness, saying anything and everything that comes to mind, without censoring. This might include confusing thoughts, ignorance, moral ambivalence, and negative personal experience with regard to this topic. Afterwards, compile a list of all the factors that makes this sexual issue so difficult.

Homework

With regard to the same topic, go over in your mind and write down the *facts* about this topic that you know, and decide whether these are sufficient for your child's age level. If not, use a resource book to learn additional facts and write them down. Include even more advanced information in order to field unexpected questions and be ready for your child's next learning level.

Give a Report

With regard to the same topic, imagine that you, as a resource teacher, have an invitation to give your child's class (pick a grade from first through fifth) a brief report on this sexual topic. You need to include the facts suitable for this grade and a few basic moral or ethical principles that should benefit children, regardless of specific religious background. Imagine a few questions that might come from the class. Read your brief report in front of a mirror.

Transfer of Learning

Imagine that in a brief discussion (which could have been in response to reading a sex education book together), you have given your child the information contained in the report. In addition, you have discussed your specific moral values and standards you expect of your child. Imagine now that you want to help your child learn how the information and values might apply in real-life situations, and to give your child practice in making good decisions.

Create and present a moral dilemma around this topic that could realistically happen to a child this age, and guide his or her thoughtful decision making with Socratic questions. For example, suppose the difficult topic you have been working on is sexual orientation (and you have already given some facts and your moral views). You might say, "What if you and your third-grade friends, during play-

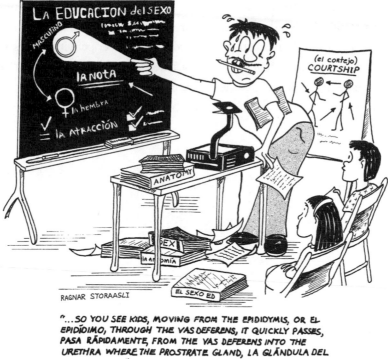

RAGNAR STORAASLI

"...SO YOU SEE KIDS, MOVING FROM THE EPIDIDYMIS, OR EL EPIDIDIMO, THROUGH THE VAS DEFERENS, IT QUICKLY PASSES, PASA RÁPIDAMENTE, FROM THE VAS DEFERENS INTO THE URETHRA WHERE THE PROSTRATE GLAND, LA GLÁNDULA DEL PROSTRATE...."

ground time, have been calling other kids queer and fag, and then one day, they call you that, and start telling other kids. What would you feel? Think? Do?" Or if the topic is early boy-girl attractions and relationships, you might say, "Suppose you're at a party with other twelve-year-old kids, and couples start to go into separate bedrooms, bathrooms, and closets to be alone, what would you be doing? What would you be thinking? Feeling? Deciding?"

Although practicing all the exercises is important for increasing your confidence, the thrust of this entire chapter should help you with your child's sex education. You have learned how to keep your child on task to achieve competence. You have discovered the reasons and routines for administering, in small doses, the vaccines consisting of sexual facts and moral guidance. This preventive approach strengthens both you and your child to cope with the next and more difficult stage. At that point, the task is to combat the serious sexual risks that come as teenagers struggle with new internal pressures as well as the external hazards of the youth culture.

6

Teaching Kids from Twelve to Seventeen

Not yet ready for intercourse with her eighteen-year-old boyfriend, a fifteen-year-old girl mentioned that she had experimented with oral sex: "No one ever said that was bad."

Omaha World Herald, Aug. 12, 1998

The stage of adolescence receives far too much bad press that doesn't reflect the lives of most teens. Contrary to popular misconceptions, teens' emotional turmoil and personal struggles are fairly moderate and certainly normal for this life stage. In spite of their grown-up appearance, mood swings, and a certain disdain for parents, they continue to need their parents' love, care, and concern. And although a teen will experience new or stronger sexual sensations, more complicated emotions, and new mental and spiritual reactions, no Jekyll-and-Hyde transformation takes place.

If we are confused about how to relate to teenagers, how to talk to them, how to inspire them, and how to set and enforce standards, a more positive attitude is in order. We don't automatically lose influence on teens' important life decisions, although we may sometimes feel out of the loop. Nevertheless, we need to recognize that our kids still need us in their lives.

Most of what I have said about parenting young children continues to apply to adolescents. We need to be present and involved in their lives, regardless of age. We need to show love, support, encouragement. We need to offer and explain moral values and standards. And we need to set limits. Overall, parenting style and communication need to change somewhat, especially for the older teen (age sixteen to seventeen) and especially with regard to sexuality. A few new attitudes and skills will go a long way in helping us have good parent-child conversations about any subject.

One very real barrier that many parents face is the lack of time and energy. Because adolescents are older and seemingly more independent, their needs can get lost in normal family stresses—parents with demanding work schedules, overextended and overburdened single parents with little physical and psychological energy, and upsetting family changes such as job changes, divorce, and remarriage. The bottom line is that many young people spend large amounts of time alone or with peers, and many are unclear about what they are and are not allowed to do. Unfortunately, these kinds of conditions can create a sense of emptiness and make sex seem an attractive and comforting way to fill the void in their hearts and souls.

Let's start this step of teaching teens about sex and morality by recalling your own adolescent experiences.

- Did you have sexual intercourse before you were eighteen?

- What was your reaction?

- How many serious dating relationships did you have during your teen years?

- How did you cope with the breakup of teenage relationships?

Your memories might elicit understanding of adolescent feelings, but empathy is not enough. For the sexual crises that today's kids face, you need knowledge, sensitivity, and clarity about the factual and moral messages that you think will help them have a good life. This chapter provides that preparation. You will gain

- Understanding of the emotional needs of adolescents and living in the "hot zone"

- Additional sexual information for carrying out your role in teaching about sex and morality for teens

- Awareness of the unique teachable moments, opportunities, and challenges

- Refined communication and interaction skills suited for teens' more personal involvement with sexual matters

- Practice opportunities for improving and perfecting these skills

Adolescents in the "Hot Zone": Needs and Characteristics

Between the ages of twelve and seventeen, young people face the central developmental task of forming a personal identity, which includes the emerging sexual self. Erik Erikson defines the challenge as the push to gain *identity* versus *identity confusion*.[1] Here's what happens with kids who are on the right track.

- They begin to get a sense of a vocational future and the effort it will take to achieve this.

- They further solidify the sexual self. This means gaining greater clarity about what it means to be a man or a woman and what their sexual orientation is, whether heterosexual, homosexual, or bisexual.

- They begin to imagine specific aspects of their future adult life, such as whether they will marry or pursue a certain overall lifestyle.

- They begin to move, by degrees, toward a confident separation from the family.

- They sense an increasing ability to manage self and take personal responsibility for their behavior.

Achieving identity is like walking a high tightrope. The challenge is to cross the precarious abyss of adolescence to reach the brink of a promising young adult life. It is a balancing act filled with risks, and many of these risks connect to sexuality. For example, consider Kevin's experience.

Kevin is sixteen and a high school sophomore. He is a fairly good student in spite of currently being afraid to attend school. He is slight in stature and build and has been teased and harassed, especially in the past year, by boys who call him "queer" and "faggot." They also physically push him around from time to time. He spends much of his time planning how to avoid these encounters and talks only occasionally to a couple of girls.

Recently his parents discovered Kevin and Carl, a twenty-year-old man, in Kevin's bedroom engaged in sexual behavior. They have forbidden Kevin to see this man and are taking him to therapy to "straighten him out." Carl thinks Kevin should come out as gay and move in with him. In the first counseling session, Kevin's father blamed his wife for Kevin's situation. He accused her of overlooking many of Kevin's effeminate behaviors since childhood because her own brother is gay.

What are Kevin's chances of gaining a positive identity and moving on to his niche in the adult world? He may fail or quit school. He faces health risks due to possible physical violence and STDs. He may prematurely enter an intimate relationship with a possibly domineering partner. He may become alienated from his parents and lose access to family emotional and financial support. He may not find healthy ways to integrate his sexual orientation into his identity. He may experience depression and try substances and sex to deaden the pain, or he may look to suicide as a solution.

The "Hot Zone"

The hot zone refers to the steamy sexual atmosphere that surrounds adolescents, with the heat and pressure coming from both within and without. The term also describes the feel of parent-child communication in which emotions can heat up in a moment and boil over into angry, hurtful, and confusing responses. Because parents recognize their teenager's obvious physical signs of sexual maturity but often don't see matching levels of emotional maturity, their reactions can be as emotionally volatile as their child's.

The child's emerging sexuality and need for sexual guidance can leave you feeling confused and embarrassed. This response may stem from worry about your child's sexual future, but unconsciously your personal sexual anxieties come into play. In the worst cases, parents begin to distance from their teenager, withdraw their personal time and involvement in their child's life, and totally avoid the duty to provide meaningful sexual and moral guidance.

What the hot zone means for teens is that the whole topic of sexuality suddenly becomes personal. Before, they took in sexual facts dispassionately, in an almost academic matter. Now these same "facts" inhabit their bodies, causing delightful sensations along with worrisome feelings. Adolescents who haven't had ongoing good communication with parents begin to feel too grown up to ask questions about sex. In addition, because their impulses might contradict early parental teachings, they may hide their deepest feelings and thoughts out of fear of losing their parents' respect.

For these reasons, teens may find sexual discussions with parents somewhat awkward and uncomfortable. Yet, as mentioned in earlier chapters, research studies show that they still want to hear parents' views, values, and advice. Because teens are in a position to act independently at this time, they need, more than ever, to know what their parents expect of them.

Parents' Role in Promoting Personal Identity

The design that the young person's personal identity takes will depend, to a large extent, on her approach to her sexual life. In other words, the threads of identity and sexuality are interwoven, and a flaw in either weakens the other. If that happens, the desired smooth, seamless fabric of identity materializes into a coarse piece filled with breaks and tears.

You need to help your kid gain a positive personal identity *and* a healthy sense of his sexuality, because both will affect his chances for a happy, meaningful life. So concerns about teenagers and sex cannot focus on morals and ethics in a narrow sense, such as whether it's right or wrong to engage in premarital sexual activity. Just as important is the question of how that behavior affects the child's overall emotional health and development—specifically, the formation of his identity.

As parents, you can guide your teen with two ethical arguments in favor of delaying intimate sexual relationships. You can say that teen sex is wrong because it is morally wrong (if that's what you believe) and explain why. You can also say that early sex is wrong or risky from the perspective of health. Then explain why: adolescents need time to form their personal identity and gain the emotional maturity to manage the risks and the meanings of a sexual relationship.

The second argument comes from the behavioral science explanation that sees the risks of early sexual activity as robbing young people of the time, focus, and opportunities that can enrich their understanding of self and relationships. This concern goes beyond the usual risks of early intercourse, which include pregnancy, disease, and emotional turmoil. Any of these unfortunate outcomes cannot only attack and possibly dismantle the fledgling identity but also may prematurely push young people out of the family nest and into adulthood—without the tools and resources to manage the new life stage.

Understanding the Risk Factors Linked to Adolescent Sexual Behavior

For reasons of both overall health and moral-ethical development, helping youth delay adolescent sexual relationships makes sense. Here you will find some clear-cut arguments for this advice that you can use in your talks with your teenager. Before going further to learn about your role in promoting this goal, review the following list summarizing the risk factors that are linked to early sexual initiation or adolescent sexual intercourse. (This does not mean that these factors *cause* the behavior.)[2] Notice that the risk factors stem from various types of influences: biological, psychological (personality, motivation), and social (friends, environment, parents, and family conditions).

- Being male

- Being African American

- Being low-income urban African American

- Early puberty (menarche, physical development, and so on)

- Early dating or steady, frequent dating

- Use of alcohol or drugs

- Daily smoking

- Driving while intoxicated

- Delinquent behavior

- Perception that friends are sexually active

- For girls, having many sexually active girlfriends

- For girls, presence of an adolescent childbearing sister

- Poor relationship with parents

- Single parent or unstable households

- Change in parents' marriage during school years

- Dating behavior of divorced mothers of adolescents
  (linked to sons' sexual activity and to daughters' sexually permissive attitudes)

The obvious challenge to you is to keep your child from whole-
sale exposure to these risks while also encouraging the conditions
that allow her to stay focused on developing a healthy identity.
Keeping your teen out of harm's way buys her time and opportunity
to grow up and become her own person. With enough time, a youth
can try out many avenues for finding her strengths, talents, and
interests. These avenues include school, special academic interests,
and extracurricular activities; hobbies; travel; relationships with
friends, family, and mentors; and participation in community life,
such as through a job, church attendance, service, and community
events and opportunities.

These varied experiences, and time to sort them out, can help
give birth to a strong sense of self and personal identity, including
the sexual self, that feels right. With this achievement, young peo-

ple then begin to imagine and pursue both short-term and long-terms goals and dreams.

Understanding the Central Role of Identity in Adolescent Sexual Decision Making

Do you wonder how your child would make a sexual decision in a particular situation (or, for that matter, how you might make such a decision)? Various researchers have explored this issue of health-related personal decision making, and, as you might expect, it is a complicated process.

Put simply, we should be concerned with whether the young person is developing a positive or negative identity. The quality of the personal identity is critically important because it is central to decision making in sexual situations (and others as well). And, vice versa, sexual decisions affect the continuing development of a teenager's identity. Recently researchers have looked closely at how the cognitive process of decision making (both conscious and unconscious) might work for adolescents.

One model proposed for adolescent decision making specifically includes the role of identity. Lilly Langer and George Warheit give central importance to a teenager's developing identity, which emerges over several years and interacts with the new tasks and responsibilities of this life stage.[3] Their account suggests all the many factors that parents should pay attention to in teaching their kids about sex and morality. Their model says that nearly *everything* (or at least a host of influences) affects the sexual decisions your teenager will make. As an example, let's apply Langer and Warheit's model to a boy.

1. His *tentative identity* operates like a central clearinghouse to make sense of all the influences that go into the decision he needs to make. (This identity includes his age; biological and psychological characteristics, such as personality, consciousness, and coping

and social skills; and his current sense of identity in terms of his abilities, future positive place in the world, growing independence, and personal responsibility for self.)

2. His still-forming identity (continuing to draw on parents, peers, and self for direction) even affects how much and what type of sexual knowledge and beliefs he will absorb from your sex education and from all other sources.

3. His knowledge and beliefs (but not only these) influence whether he will even get into sexual situations that call for a decision. (These include his beliefs about himself and his future, which are still developing through his interactions with parents, peers, and the social environment.)

4. If he does get into a sexual situation, then he has to process, through the clearinghouse of his tentative identity, the immediate cues in that situation that push him to behave in a certain way.

5. In the specific situation, many emotions, thoughts, and behaviors are happening, often unconsciously, all at once (especially if you or school programs haven't given him practice in sexual decision making). He draws on his knowledge and beliefs, and figures out which influence to allow to direct his thinking (parents, peers, or self); he begins to weigh his physical and sexual needs in the moment, his psychological needs and motivations in the moment, and the social pressure in the moment (such as from his partner, a party situation where everyone is pairing off, and so on) to arrive at a decision.

6. All these elements go back into some kind of process of self-analysis within and through the identity. Depending on all the aforementioned factors, he may or may not bring much consciousness to his decision, evaluating and applying knowledge and beliefs in relation to needs. Some of the beliefs would be about himself, his partner, the meaning of sex, its place in relationships, and what is right or moral conduct.

7. His decision then produces a specific behavior (such as to engage in sex or not, to use a condom or not, and so on).

8. The behavior he chooses and the attitudes that follow it *continue to contribute to his still-forming identity*. In other words, the choices themselves in that situation bring about new biological, psychological, and social factors that will continue to influence the knowledge and beliefs that he will absorb into his identity.

This model of decision making supports the stance that I have maintained throughout the book. We need to put effort into strengthening children for this adolescent stage when life becomes very complicated. One sex talk at the beginning of puberty doesn't do it. Such strengthening can only happen gradually through all the nurturing, information, and guidance that we give through each stage of development. With this approach to sex education, we can have some influence on how our child will make sexual and other life decisions.

That said, how do you proceed on a day-to-day basis to teach and guide your adolescent child? First, keep your eye on your son or daughter's developing identity and whether it's moving in a wholesome direction. Second, given that early or intense sexual relationships can hinder the development of identity, you can follow two broad strategies that help promote conscious decision making, as suggested in Langer and Warheit's model.

1. With a young adolescent (ages twelve to fifteen), make it clear that you expect delay of involvement in intimate sexual activity, especially intercourse, and provide the supervision and family rules that give this expectation meaning and priority. The young person who has time to form a healthy identity will have that identity in place for making more conscious sexual decisions during the later teens.

2. With the older teen, foster a rich understanding of the sexual self, the emotional aspects of sex, and the deeper meanings of love, committed relationships, and marriage and how these play out in real life. These meanings too become part of your child's identity

and beliefs, thus helping the young person make more conscious sexual decisions that include, besides all the risks, the meanings of the sex to both partners and their lives.

These two strategies are interrelated, and the division is simply a matter of focus. Even with older teens, you can still talk about various reasons for delaying, or deciding not to have, sexual intercourse. And with the younger teen, you could also be talking about your values about the deeper or emotional meanings of sex and relationships. The following section offers practical details and specific sexual information that can be part of parent-teen discussions about life in the hot zone.

The Role of Parents in Teaching About Sex and Morality

You have two roles to carry out in your adolescent's sex education and moral guidance. First, make sure that your teenager, during this stage, gets the full facts about sexuality. Do this by seeing whether his or her school offers full coverage and by supplementing that information (whether it is complete or not) with additional resources that you personally give your child, especially in the form of age-appropriate books. (See "Sex Education Resources" in the Resources.) Your active involvement in the sexual information that your child gets gives you a critical entry point for talking about sex. Second, approach the topics in ways that school programs and books cannot: talk about some of the more sensitive, private, or controversial aspects of sexuality and about your family's moral values and standards. Remember, personal and moral beliefs, in addition to factual knowledge, are important in the adolescent decision-making process described earlier.

With adolescents, we have to go beyond the brief facts and clear-cut moral guidelines that worked for the preteen. Because they are refining their ability to reason, think in abstractions, and imagine hypothetical situations, teens want to know the basis for information and advice. Whereas I favor simply invoking parental authority with young children, rigid or dramatic directives don't encourage adolescents to learn how to think critically in decision making. They need practice in sorting out reasons and preparing for the day when their own self-directed identity will guide their choices. We give them that practice when our talks include reasons and explanations.

In this section, I am not going to explain specific sexual facts. You make sure your child gets these—with thorough explanations, diagrams, and other learning tools—through school sex education, talks with you, and the books you provide. By the facts I mean sexual anatomy, physiology, development, and functioning; sexual behaviors (abstinence, masturbation, intercourse, and so on); relationships, dating, and marriage; pregnancy, childbirth, contraception, and abortion; STDs; sexual identity and orientation; family life and parenting; sex and the media; and sex and the law, including pornography, prostitution, and sexual offenses.

There are good reasons to count on school programs and books to provide the full facts of sexuality. First, these methods can deliver sexual material in a comprehensive and more or less "cool" academic context that can bring some balance to the hot zone of adolescence. The complete facts are essential to correct sexual myths and misinformation that youths face in daily life. Second, the facts offer a basic safety net for the tightrope walk toward identity. A teen who flounders and gets into premature sexual activity may need to draw on factual knowledge, such as the use of contraception and condoms, to cushion the fall and prevent serious damage.

What I cover here is information that will give you a rationale (which assumes an understanding of sexual facts) for the two parental strategies. That is, it offers reasons for (1) why young teens should delay intimate sexual activity and (2) why older teens should learn more about the deeper meanings of sex and how it affects the self and relationships in adult life. Moral and ethical threads are also interwoven with these ideas (you should add your unique moral views as well). These thoughts encourage teens to clarify their values, learn how to talk rationally about sex, and make decisions that they can implement and take responsibility for. Finally, you will also see how to include in your talks the *positive* aspects of sexuality, not only dangers and warnings.

Rationale for Delaying Sexual Relationships

During the 1980s, Sharon Thompson conducted in-depth interviews with four hundred teenage girls regarding their reactions to their first experience with sexual intercourse.[4] Many girls gave similar accounts of their reasons and reactions.

> *"Maybe I just did it unconsciously."*
>
> *"I didn't know, you know, that a guy would put his penis in me like that."*
>
> *"One minute here, the next minute it was there. It happened. That was it."*
>
> *"The pain was like I couldn't stand it."*
>
> *"I didn't realize basically what I got myself into."*
>
> *"I don't think I was emotionally capable of handling it at the time."*
>
> *"It wasn't that I didn't like it. It was just kind of a letdown."*
>
> *"There was nothing I liked about it."*
>
> *"He wasn't supposed to penetrate. . . ."*

These comments suggest several common threads in the girls' reactions. They denied conscious choice. They were not prepared for the reality of naked bodies, sex organs, and the mechanics of sex. It happened very fast. It was often painful, boring, or a letdown. Whereas some girls revealed that they waited a while before having sex again, they often had the same stunned reaction several times before becoming more conscious and responsible by obtaining contraception. In contrast to this group, other girls in the study who were more conscious about the decision to have sex, who planned for it, and who were tuned into their own desire recalled their first intercourse as a positive experience.

Arguments for Delay Preventing a Bad Sexual Experience Thompson's study and others have shown that when girls suggest the ideal age for intercourse, they usually give a higher age than that of their own sexual initiation. These results definitely support the rationale that a girl should delay intercourse until she is old enough to both "know" and emotionally process information about sex, boys, her own identity and wishes, her own sexual interest, risks, and protection. She should also wait until she is able to be more conscious in the choice to say no or yes to sex. This degree of emotional maturity takes time to develop, especially for girls, who get a lot of messages to be agreeable and passive in relationships.

What about boys and their first intercourse experience? Several research findings suggest that boys too are often "in over their heads" in that experience. For example, boys know much less about sex in general than girls. They have also reported, with regret, that during first intercourse, they didn't know what they were doing, focused only on their own pleasure, and didn't understand anything about a girl's needs. In addition, boys often don't feel in charge of themselves or a sexual situation: 32 percent of *late* adolescent boys, compared to only 9 percent of girls, felt unable or very uncertain about being able to refuse a sexual advance by a partner. Although boys typically have a positive response to intercourse, one study found that more males than females engaged in unwanted intercourse. And when that happened, their reasons were to prove themselves, live up to expectations, and be popular. Even college-age men feel they can't easily say no to sex, can't talk about sex in a sexual situation with a partner, and wouldn't be able stop intercourse in a situation where they lacked protection.[5]

The point is that young adolescent boys, just like girls, are not mature enough to understand and manage the risks and complexities that go with sexual intercourse. Besides facing the possibility of disease and pregnancy, they also risk having a mediocre or unsuccessful sexual experience for themselves and most certainly for their partner. In my study of adolescent sexuality, 25 percent of boys said that, following their first intercourse experience, they did not feel "sexually satisfied." For girls, 72 percent said they did not feel sexually satisfied.[6] Again, boys hear a lot about the risks of pregnancy and disease. What they also need to hear is that sexual intercourse will be more satisfying and meaningful if they are mature enough to understand themselves, their partner, and all that goes with this intimate act. They need to develop the self-assurance to make the conscious choice to say no or yes to sex.

Arguments for Delay Promoting a Good Sexual Experience These findings about boys and girls give new arguments for advising teens to delay intimate sexual relationships. You can point out the positive benefits of waiting, not merely give warnings to avoid negative outcomes. You might put it this way: "Your sexuality is going to be with you for your lifetime. It can be part of the wonderful adventure of life or like a bad dream that you want to forget. If you give yourself time to grow up and wait to have a sexual relationship when you're old enough, it will likely be more pleasurable and meaningful, and it won't leave bad memories and feelings. These can affect your future chances for a satisfying sex life."

This rationale does not deny other strong reasons for not engaging in intercourse (risk of pregnancy, disease, loss of reputation, emotional turmoil, moral viewpoints, and so on). But it captures a truth about pleasure and the meaning of sex that your teen may not hear from any other source.

In this approach, you have to be appropriately personal by saying that you advise the delay because you want your child to have a fulfilling sexual future. This means you acknowledge that a good sex life is something of value and that sexual pleasure is legitimate. Having this more personal kind of conversation is easier said than done. Many parents can barely talk about sexual facts and are squeamish about delving into moral issues. Yet consider how this parental message can reflect sincere caring for your child's future: "I hope the first time you have sex will be exciting, pleasurable, and meaningful."

Kids know that sex is about pleasure, and parents who can briefly and properly allow this point gain credibility with their child. In addition, the "pleasure principle" can also be a part of your approach to other moral or spiritual dimensions of sex. Finally, all the messages in the world about reasons for delaying sex will be mere fluff if you don't put parental authority behind the advice by setting limits on your young teen's activities—such as dating and unsupervised time with friends at home, parties, and so on—and monitoring those activities.

"Heart to Heart" with Young Teens: Benefits of Delaying Sexual Relationships

We've looked in some detail at a central reason for youth to delay intimate sexual activity, namely, that sex can be more exciting, enjoyable, pleasurable, fulfilling, and meaningful if you're mature enough to know what you're doing, to make a conscious choice, and to do it for yourself and your partner with mutual care, honesty, and responsibility.

This rationale applies to both boys and girls. For too long, sexual advice to girls has centered on boys' desire and girls' responsibility to keep a lid on it. This message denies girls' sexual desire and their right to sexual pleasure, or treats these as a sign of poor morals. Stereotypes of hypermasculinity and hyperfemininity feed off each other, and change has to begin with both boys and girls. Teens, just like adults, have much to gain by regarding each other as people with unique qualities, not as stereotyped gender symbols. If, by nature and nurture, the sexes do tend to differ in their approach to sex (men more focused on the physical aspects of sexual pleasure, women on its emotional connection), then we should help teens (who will be adults soon) capitalize on the differences and learn from each other in ways that may enrich sex and intimacy for both.

Let's explore some additional benefits that teens can reap from delaying sex—besides the fact that it can lead to better sex. Remember that the underlying assumption of this chapter is that teenagers need time to form a healthy identity because this is crucial to their entire future well-being and happiness. Although I couch the following ideas in language that you could use with a teen, don't look on these thoughts as sermons or speeches. Ideally, you and your teen would have many give-and-take talks—which might be brief, passing interactions—that could naturally give rise to these topics.

Make a point of having a dialogue when you and your teen talk about the sexual matters I offer here. Obviously, you might also want to spell out more clearly your ethical message and whether this comes from religious or other philosophical beliefs. My remarks speak directly to the child and, at times, include useful information about teens in general. Notice that the focus often moves intentionally from teenagers to adults to give young people a taste of the realities of adult life.

Becoming Your Own Person You need time to learn about, appreciate, and value yourself, for who you are and what you can become, as your own person, regardless of whether you have a relationship, lots of friends, or a certain appearance. When kids don't like themselves for the person they are and are becoming, they often latch on to others, a group, or a particular person to make them feel worthwhile. The more you become your own person, the more you will know what you want in your daily life and make choices that are right for you.

Friendship You need time to learn more about friendships, time to make and be friends with both boys and girls, and learn what makes a real friend, such as trust, caring, shared interests, honest communication, and loyalty. Experts tell us that boys find it hard to make deep friendships with either boys or girls and that girls often wound others with words, including their friends. Understanding friendship will help you figure out what qualities you would want in a serious love relationship and improve your chances of making a good choice when you enter marriage or a committed relationship. Learning about friendships will give you experience in understanding people and their motives and help you learn how to judge situations and a person's character.

Early Sexual Attractions and Feelings You need time to learn about what you and your friends are feeling as you start growing up. Teenagers naturally start to have strong emotions, attractions, and interest in relationships. Boys and girls differ in some ways but are the same in others. You can enjoy these feelings, but also try to step back and see how some motives and actions can get out of hand. The problem is the tendency for both boys and girls to want a partner as somewhat of a trophy. Girls sometimes become obsessed with the idea of having a boyfriend or getting a boy to go with them (and getting this and talking about it with other girls probably gives their ego a boost). Boys sometimes focus on girls as sex objects who will bring them sexual release (and getting this or just talking about "scoring" probably gives their ego a boost).

These may be fairly typical reactions for young people just discovering their sexuality. But some kids get stuck with these limited ideas and never move on. They never come to a deeper appreciation of themselves or of the opposite sex or of what makes for a good sexual or love relationship. Without this, people can stay stuck and continue having selfish or self-centered reasons for being in a relationship, which is like using the partner for their own selfish purposes. This behavior follows many kids right into adulthood; they keep doing the same pattern and then wondering why they don't find a lasting, fulfilling love relationship.

Unhealthy Patterns in Relationships When teenagers start intense dating relationships too early, both boys and girls can become almost addicted to the need to have a relationship. They may accept and stay in a relationship, regardless of whether it is healthy or makes them happy. Here's why. Early boy-girl relationships cause strong warm, exciting feelings, which feel good. But if your partner wants out or a relationship ends, you can be left with very bad feelings that you're not emotionally ready to handle. One way that some kids deal with their pain is to quickly latch on to another relationship. What this means is that they don't learn to deal in healthy ways with their disappointment and learn from their experience. In other words, they don't learn to go slower, build a real friendship, hold off on sex until they are mature enough for this experience. Without learning something from experience, they just go on following the same pattern, right into adult life. This is the same pattern that causes adult men and women to jump from one relationship to another. They never learn that another person cannot give them value. You have to love yourself and feel worthwhile as an individual before you can share your life in a healthy way with another person.

A Girl Thing, a Guy Thing You need time to learn how a boy and a girl might experience a sexual situation with each other quite differently. Most of what goes on is unconscious unless you are mature enough to know your deep feelings or to talk during sex with your partner. Girls often feel emotionally close and in love, and they want to engage in sex to please a partner and strengthen the relationship. They may even imagine a long-term commitment, even though they are still teenagers. Boys often do not feel the same emotional connection, although they may like or feel love for their partner. They may see sex as part of their experience in growing up and not even imagine a deep emotional commitment until much later in life, when they consciously begin taking that step.

There's a lot of misunderstanding between boys and girls when they have sex without the ability and maturity to be honest and talk about what it means. Kids who can't talk to each other and don't know their own or their partner's intentions are not old enough for sex. Because many adults can't do this either, they often never create a meaningful and satisfying sexual relationship.

Rationale for Learning About the Deeper Meanings of Love and Sex

Many parents sense that young people need guidance that goes beyond the simple prescription, Be abstinent until marriage and all will be well. For too long we have wistfully imagined that the younger generation would absorb from the term *marriage* alone the Nirvana of what a love relationship is all about. We often simply assume that they will discover on their own, without explanation, what to look for in a lifetime mate, how to decide on that commitment, and what it takes to sustain a marriage.

Why would we expect this when young people know that half of marriages end in divorce, and many of them have lived through the breakup of their own parents' marriage? How will they learn about the deeper meanings of an intimate love relationship if we as parents do not tell them? Even if we have not achieved a lasting love relationship in our own lives, we have to find honest and sincere ways to tell them about this value.

A recent story in the *Washington Post* reported on a situation in which thirteen- and fourteen-year-olds from a mostly upper-income suburban community were engaging in oral sex. School and health officials suggested that this sexual activity reflected a "disturbing pattern of middle schoolers who are adopting an 'anything but intercourse' approach to sex. Eager to avoid pregnancy and hold on to virginity, an increasing number of teens are engaging in oral sex."[7] Such early initiation into sex and the casual attitude toward oral sex suggest that these young people were acting on messages from the media, friends, and their own adolescent sexual urges and curiosity.

We can wonder if the parents ever clearly told these kids that intimate sexual activity is part of marriage or a serious relationship.

Did the parents tell them that young people need time to grow up before they can forge such a deep relationship? Even if these teens had heard these messages, we should still wonder why they gave them so little thought or didn't worry about "getting in trouble" with parents or the school. In today's world, when a lot of adults themselves seem to pursue the cult of youth and all that goes with it, young people may not take parents' advice very seriously—if any is given. Clearly, as argued throughout this book, meaningful sexual and moral guidance for children is much more than sexual facts, warnings, or a single moral guideline, regardless of whether it's "wait till marriage" or "use protection."

At some point in researching and writing this book, I heard an interesting analogy (I don't remember the source) between the images the media present for both automobiles and sex. It went like this.

> What if your entire knowledge of cars came from television, movies, and video games? You would see images appealing to looks, style, innovation, status, excitement, power, and success. Then come other scenes suggesting that cars are all about the high drama of chases, crashes, and explosions without real consequences for the people in the story. From these depictions, would you gain an understanding of the mechanisms that make a car run, a rational basis for comparing different models, costs compared to value, the benefits of function and long-term ownership versus trading often, the importance of safe driving, requirements for insurance, and benefits of regular maintenance and repair service?

Enough said! The analogy to media images of sex is obvious. If parents don't let their kids know about the facts of sex and the deeper human meanings and consequences of sexual relationships, who will?

Connecting with Older Teens:
The Deeper Meanings of Sex, Self, and Relationships

If you're wondering exactly what older teens need to hear from parents, recall that I am assuming they are getting the full facts about sexuality and protection through school sex education programs and books and discussions you provide. That said, we will explore other, more personal topics that parents and schools usually bypass.

The message to delay intimate sexual relationships is still appropriate (based on your moral values, on the importance of allowing time for identity to develop, and so on). But parents need to also recognize that older teens are becoming more independent and will likely have more freedom as they show the ability to handle their independence responsibly. Many teenagers begin to date, with their parents' approval, on a more or less regular basis by age sixteen or seventeen, and some will have rather steady dating relationships. These may last several months or continue for longer periods.

It's at this point that parents begin to wonder if their child has become sexually active. They may worry but not quite know what to do, especially if they haven't talked about sex and relationships before. Even under these circumstances, rather than simply worry, you can use this new stage of dating to explore your son or daughter's understanding of sex. These situations demand sensitivity, because teens want you to respect their privacy and personal boundaries.

Because we know that many older teens have dating and other relationships that may call for sexual decisions, we need to consider what kind of parent-child talks, beyond the facts of sex, would help. There are two major moral and ethical concerns to plan for: (1) Is my child gaining an appreciation of the nature of intimate love and sexual relationships and an understanding of his or her own needs for a close relationship? and (2) Will my teenager have this moral mind-set before facing the decision about engaging in a sexual relationship?

The following remarks speak to teenagers directly and are simply examples of what you might say in give-and-take dialogues and during various talks. Do not think of these ideas as speeches or lectures to deliver in a single breath.

Real-Life Sex and Real Emotions People feel many complicated emotions in a real marriage or real sexual relationship, compared to the romance and fantasies of the movies. Feelings can range from ecstatic to betrayed. Many kids have said that even though they knew the facts of sex, they weren't prepared for the emotional part of a sexual relationship. Here's what they mean. When you have sex with a person, you already have some feelings for the person and about yourself, but these get much more complicated afterwards. In sex, because you expose a lot of your self—and not just your body— you begin to expect something in return for sharing yourself in this intimate way. People often expect that the relationship will continue and that both partners will show equal interest, affection, emotional involvement, trust, dependency, shared understandings, and love for each other. Sex often makes partners think a lot about each other, look forward to being together, and expect to have sex on a regular basis.

In both marriage and sexual relationships, partners are never exactly on the same wavelength. They may have different needs and ideas with regard to feelings, sex, and their relationship. Misunderstandings happen a lot because we all carry around fantasies in our heads about what we want from our partner. When people have a strong love and commitment to each other, they intend to stick around and try to work out these differences.

When this doesn't work and our emotional bond seems weak, we can easily start to feel hurt, disappointed, lonely, rejected, used, even betrayed. Both the ecstatic feelings of connection, excitement, and pleasure as well as the bad feelings are intense. This is a lot for people to handle—teenagers or adults, single or married. It will help if you can learn all of this a little at a time, so you'll know what real life is like. It takes time to become mature enough to enjoy the good times and roll with the bad.

The Nitty-Gritty of Sex, Sex Organs, and Bodies If you're going to have sex, you need to be ready for the mechanics of sex. This means naked bodies, your partner seeing and touching your private parts, and coordinating what you both want to do. This includes the practical matters relating to birth control and protection against diseases (these issues don't magically go away with marriage). This means making sure that you have prepared ahead of time, know how to use your chosen methods, and are confident about handling any mishaps (like a condom that breaks), and so on.

Carrying out all these responsibilities takes some getting used to. Some adults, married or single, never get comfortable with this part of sex. Some women don't like to let their partners see their bodies, or they worry about their appearance instead of being able to enjoy the sexual relationship. And both adult men and women, married or single, often make the mistake of failing to plan for birth control and protection. You have to have high self-esteem and emotional maturity to deal with and enjoy the physical aspects of real sex.

Privacy and Real Sex People often don't realize how much of themselves they show and share in sex. Afterwards you may think about this and naturally assume that both of you will respect the privacy and specialness of what you shared together in those intimate moments. Teenagers who aren't mature enough to have sex violate this trust by talking to others, often in great detail, about the sexual relationship, their partner's body, their behaviors, their reactions, and so on. Think about whether this is what you would want your partner to do within hours or days after you had sex with each other.

You see and hear these "blow-by-blow" accounts on television or in movies like they're a big joke. You also hear them in school bathrooms, locker rooms, hallways, and among friends talking at the mall, slumber parties, and so on. People who are mature enough to have sex realize that sex is a private, meaningful act that involves "flesh-and-blood" human beings with feelings. If partners have worries or concerns after sex, they shouldn't broadcast these to friends, acquaintances, and eavesdroppers in the next booth at Wendy's. This doesn't mean you shouldn't talk to anyone. Partners who care about each other and are mature enough to have sex should talk privately about any worries or about their experience with each other. But if that doesn't seem like a good idea, then they could talk privately with a trusted friend or a parent.

True Choice and Real Sex Many teenagers, and some adults, get into a sexual relationship in an unconscious or impulsive way. This is not the route to a satisfying, meaningful sexual experience. Instead of the conscious, thinking part of the mind making a true choice, feelings, impulses, or perhaps alcohol or drugs are in charge. These people may fool themselves into thinking the sex was spontaneous and just happened or that their feelings of love were responsible. Here are some of those kinds of emotional or wrong reasons for having sex. See if you've heard them before: I did it because I was bored, curious, too excited to stop, depressed, pressured, under the influence; I did it because I felt obligated to my partner, wanted to get a partner, wanted to keep a partner, wanted to be popular, wanted to impress my friends, and on and on.

So what's involved in a true choice? First of all, if it's a true choice, the whole sexual experience will be better, more meaningful, more pleasurable. What if you're "in love"? Here are some ideas about the "right" reasons that show a person has some understanding of love, relationships, and self and has given rational thought to the possibility of having sex. "Love" or a deep caring means a lot of things.

- You value and care about both yourself and the other person equally.

- You know, value, and respect each other.

- You know your own needs and believe you have healthy motives.

- You feel attraction to and desire for *this particular person*.

- You believe the sex is right for the relationship and will not harm it.

- You are honest with yourself and your partner about what the sex and your relationship mean to each of you.

- You can also tell if this is a true choice if your "right" reasons allow you to act in a responsible way.

- Your choice is in line with your sexual and life values.

- You and your partner can communicate about sex and have planned for birth control and protection against disease.

- You can handle any outcomes of the sexual relationship (including more complicated emotions and continued expectations for intercourse).

- You believe the sex will not interfere with your life goals and those of your partner.

These are just starters. You need to have a lot of things in place before you have sex. In a marriage or committed relationship, partners feel secure that they can meet all these conditions. Because they have made a true choice, they then feel free to be their true selves during sex, which helps make the experience satisfying for both partners. Even in marriage, all of this doesn't always come together. So it's a lot more complicated if you're not married.

You need time to learn all the steps involved in making a true, rational choice. If you're seriously thinking about having sex, I hope you will take your time and give a lot of thought to this list. It can help you and your partner see whether you have this kind of honest, caring relationship and can take on the responsibilities that go with sex. This is one way to figure out if you are ready for a sexual relationship, and making a conscious decision will improve your chances for making it a good experience. Remember, I'm always willing to talk more about this any time you want or about any decisions you're thinking about.

When Relationships End Kids your age know at some level that, no matter how intense the relationship is and how much energy they put into it, teenage relationships will end (and, unfortunately, many marriages as well). That tells you about how difficult relationships are. It also tells you that you will probably have several important relationships that will end before you decide on a deep or formal commitment, such as marriage. This is a good reason to go slowly with relationships. Make them positive by becoming friends with your partner. Don't rush to turn them into complicated emotional and sexual relationships before you're ready to put your heart, soul, and energy into this. Enjoy these relationships for the good feelings, fun, adventure, and learning that you get from them.

Even when they're not sexual, it will hurt when they end. Then you need to cope with your pain, remember the good, value the whole experience for what you learned and how you grew, and change yourself if changes are needed. Do the same if the relationship was sexual, and evaluate what you learned from that experience too, and use the new learning in your future life. These and any other concerns are things you can talk to me about. You don't need to deal with your hurts or worries all on your own.

———————

So far, you have learned that in the hot zone of adolescence, young people begin to take steps into the larger world, and adults need to help them pace the journey. Part of that trip is the tightrope walk toward a personal identity and claiming the sexual self. Teens need time to reach this destination before they risk getting bogged down in sexual problems and premature adult responsibilities.

You can help by making sure they have the full facts about sexuality and clear moral guidelines. Here you saw some good reasons for delaying involvement in intimate sexual relationships; you can include them in your parent-child talks. You also got ideas on how to talk about the complications and the deeper meanings surrounding sex, love, emotional intimacy, and marriage. The next step is to tune into and create opportunities for these personal talks.

Teachable Moments, Opportunities, and Challenges

The nature of teenage life furnishes plenty of opportunities for you to talk with your kid about sex, yet broaching the subject in the hot zone can be intimidating. You should both initiate sexual discussions and use naturally occurring situations to keep sexual matters as part of normal conversation.

Initiating Sexual Discussions

Taking the lead is usually easier with younger teens because they expect that you will continue with the sex education you started prior to puberty. Older youth, because of more intense sexual feelings, dating, or being in relationships, tend to become more private and somewhat guarded about sharing too much or asking for information. The ease or difficulty, however, with a child of any age often depends on whether you and child have had good communication in the past, especially with regard to sex.

With a young teen, you can definitely take the lead by planning to talk about his school sex education program and the new books that you give him. But you will need to adapt your approach. For example, you are not likely be sitting with your thirteen-year-old at bedtime reading a sex book.

Consider the following ideas that go beyond simply giving a book to your child and reminding her to read it. (This basic effort would not be a waste. Simply giving teenagers a book on sex, even without talking about it, is a step that most parents don't take.) But by reading this book you are preparing to do that and much more.

First, buy a good sex education book directed to teens that is comprehensive enough to see your child through the entire adolescent stage. (See "Sex Education Resources" in the Resources.) By now you appreciate that full sexual information is necessary, especially in view of the extensive sexual content that comes kids' way from television, the Internet, and friends. For example, a lot of teens watch daytime talk shows and cable movies. (MTV's *Loveline* is a favorite, but this show at least provides expert professional answers to questions about sex, along with a lot of humor as well.) Giving a book on sexuality sends the positive message that you care about your child's future, that you believe knowing sexual facts is important, and that people in your family can talk about sex.

Second, become very familiar with the book's contents before you pass it on (more on this later). You want to know that the messages are factual, healthy, and constructive, and exactly which sections speak strongly to your values or would make for a good discussion.

Third, present the book with enthusiasm and a brief explanation:

> This is a really good book on sex that I got for you. It has information on everything you need to know for now and as you get older too. So as you're reading it I want us to talk about it. Not just a big talk but just as things come up. There are some things in there that are really important that I want to be sure we talk about. You know I wish I had had a book like this. Did I ever tell you how my parents gave me my sex education? . . . I want to make sure you know everything you need to know about sex because this will definitely help you in

life. Life and sex are really complicated today, much
more so than when I was growing up.

Being familiar with the book is essential because it becomes an
entry point for having follow-up discussions. This is how you *create*
opportunities. So before you hand it over, take a few notes on specific topics or the author's treatment of a topic that you want to talk
about or that you think will engage your teenager. Then use these
notes (perhaps from time to time) as openers to invite a discussion.

For your opening remarks, start with a personal reaction rather
than a question that a kid could ignore. For example:

- I thought the explanation about sex stereotypes was
  good.

- I wish I had known some of what it says about love
  and marriage when I was a teenager.

- Let's go over the important stuff about STDs (or other
  topics). Kids often have questions about this. I want to
  make sure you understand this information. It's really
  important. HIV and AIDS are life-and-death matters.
  This is a matter of your life we're talking about.

You can also create opportunities to talk about sex by following
up on your child's learning about sexuality in school classes or a sex
education course. Learn how such courses as biology, human development, and family living cover sexual topics. Ideally, teachers
would give assignments requiring students to talk to parents about
selected issues. If this doesn't happen, however, you can make the
first move.

Rather than asking a general question, such as how the class is
going, raise a specific question in order to encourage a response. If
you don't get one, briefly give your thoughts on the topic and
explain why you think it's a good idea for parents and kids to talk

about the school programs. Keep these efforts positive and light-hearted, even if your child seems uninterested. For example, "I'd really like to hear about what you're learning and some of the assignments. I could probably learn something myself." Remember, you can always come back with the simple and humorous reminder that providing sex education is a parental duty: "I don't want the Child Welfare Department coming around and saying that I am neglecting my kids and not giving them good care." If you get great resistance, you might say, "I would prefer that you and I talk about what you're learning so that I don't have to look stupid by asking your teacher at the next parent-teacher conference."

Another way that you can take the initiative is to tune into a new stage or new events in your child's life and use these as an opportunity for an updated discussion about sex. Think about ways to find a bridge between what you want to talk about now and perhaps some prior situation when you dealt with sex. For example, you may have had an extensive talk with your daughter at age ten or eleven about getting her period, but you now want to give her more information. Consider any new developments as a basis to initiate your talk. For example, if she is planning to go to the co-ed sleep-over at the school following eighth-grade graduation, use this event: "I can't believe we haven't updated your knowledge about sex in the past two years. I think we should talk and figure out some more things that you need to know since you are about to go into high school." There could be any number of such transitions or events: a birthday, a crush, a school trip away from parents, a vacation, changing schools, starting to date, changing neighborhoods, and so on.

To repeat a point made earlier, you should take the initiative with confidence because research tells us that the large majority of kids want to talk to their parents. Even if your child seems resistant or nonchalant, consider this part of the normal "cool" attitude of teens and don't take it personally. Continuing the effort sends the message that you are interested and willing to talk. The next time, your child may be in a more receptive mood.

Making the Most of Teachable Moments

You can also introduce sexual content as part of naturally occurring activities in life. These include the various situations mentioned in earlier chapters, such as commenting on or discussing media portrayals of sex, sexual issues in the news, and the lives of family or friends (relationships, engagements, marriage, pregnancy, divorce, and so on).

Besides these, the social life of the typical teen should spark discussions due to the need for your approval and monitoring of their activities. These interactions might easily present opportunities for talks about sex or relationships as a natural part of talking about the family's rules, for example:

- Who can or cannot be in the family home when you are gone

- What is allowed in regard to hanging out with groups of friends, pairing up, dating alone, and steady or serious dating

- Reasons for a curfew

- Restrictions on television, movies, the Internet, and so on

- Why you insist on meeting and getting to know your child's friends and dates

- Why you want details on proposed parties, concerts, sleepovers, and other social activities

Any time you see red flags signaling imminent risk in a teenager's behavior, it is time to initiate a more focused serious discussion. If your child shows evidence of any of the risk factors linked to early intercourse (such as alcohol use, friends who are sexually active or pregnant, or truancy from school) or you sense that something is amiss, follow your instinct and bring up your concerns. Other worrisome issues to explore include your child's having older dating partners (which is most likely to happen with girls), violating family rules, making last-minute changes in social plans, being reluctant to give details about activities, and exhibiting noticeable negative changes in behavior and mood.

Regardless of what triggers your sexual discussions, avoid preaching and warning. Do your best to have a rational, thoughtful, give-and-take dialogue; ask about your child's understanding and views of the sexual topic; and include your wish for him or her to have a good life during adolescence and in the future. Keep in mind that the content and tone of your talks will likely differ for younger versus older teens. Now go on to learn about the communication skills that can help make these parent-teen interactions positive and effective.

Parent Communication and Interaction Skills

What would you say if your teenager tossed out any of the following one-liners?

> "Meredith is all bent out of shape because I wouldn't give her my honor society pin [or football or track letter] to wear on a chain."
>
> "Every time we go out we always have to do what Dylan wants to do."
>
> "Cassie wants me to call her every evening as soon as I get home from school."
>
> "I think I'm going to break up with Rick."
>
> "Is there a test to find out if people are gay?"

Any one of these remarks offers a chance for a meaningful parent-child talk. But before spelling out some communication skills that can make such a talk happen, I will remind you of certain natural parental tendencies to avoid. I call them the five P's, and they can stifle dialogue within seconds. For example, consider how the teen-

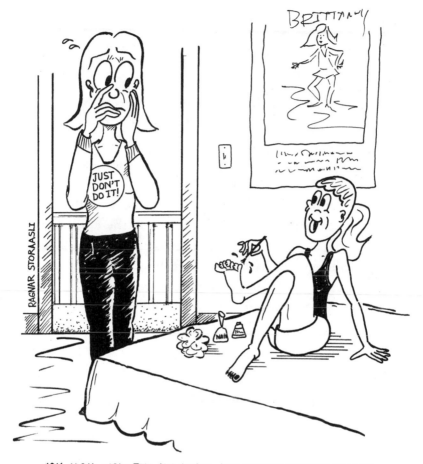

"OK, MOM, NOW TELL ME AGAIN ABOUT THAT 'SUMMER OF LOVE'
BACK IN THE SIXTIES."

ager making each of the comments here might react to these parental responses:

Premature judging	"That girl is just too pushy. You knew that from the beginning."
Pronouncements	"You should speak up for yourself."
Predictions	"You'll end up letting women walk all over you."

Pussyfooting   "Oh, now, you two will work things out."

Preaching   "Questions like that are way out of line in
           this house."

Aside from avoiding these conversation killers, what *does* work? Previously I have offered guidelines for effective communication, such as for initiating sexual discussions with your partner or spouse to resolve a sexual concern (Chapter One). Many of these communication skills also apply in talking with teenagers.

As you consider the skills discussed in this section, think about your ability to learn and use them. Not all of these will fit every topic or situation, or the personality and age of your child. If your teenager willingly pours out details or feelings about a personal situation, you may simply need to listen for a while to get a sense of where the conversation is going.

General Communication Guidelines for All Sexual Discussions

Throughout this book, I have offered various suggestions for parent-child sexual discussions. The summary here serves as a good review before going onto the next section, which covers the specific communication skills that will help you carry out these guidelines.

1. Adjust your communication style to your child's age, knowledge about sexuality, temperament, and other special needs.

2. Put balance in your overall approach, so that your remarks include the positive dimensions of sexuality and affirming messages as well as risks and responsibilities.

3. Maintain a calm, nondefensive stance, regardless of any initial shock or embarrassment you feel due to the nature of the sexual topic.

4. Maintain an attitude of respect and caring for your child, even when disagreeing or giving rules and setting limits.

5. Encourage dialogue and give-and-take. Ask for your child's understanding or view of the sexual topic. You need not dominate the conversation.

6. Explore and raise issues in a way that encourages your child to think about decisions and how to make them.

7. Take cues from your child to gauge when the conversation should come to a close.

8. End on a positive note, no matter how awkward or difficult the talk may have become, and clearly say that you look forward to more discussions.

9. Let your child know to bring any concerns or questions to you as his or her life changes, gets more complicated, or brings problems.

Important Communication Skills

Parents often wonder how to respond to a sexual question or situation so as to get the conversation under way and to keep it going. The following skills are especially important when dealing with a teenager's personal situation or problem, but they also apply to any type of sexual discussion or, for that matter, any topic.

1. During all stages of the talk, listen for what your child is sharing, asking, or needing. Listening closely will help you avoid the five P's and enable you to discover what the conversation will be about.

2. Reflect what you think your child might be feeling or thinking, tuning in to both negative and positive feelings. "Sounds like you're frustrated [bummed out, worried, confused, pretty thrilled, excited]." "It sounds like you have some questions about homosexuality."

3. Explore as needed with open-ended questions that pick up on what your teenager said, but don't interrogate or probe for personal details. For example, for some of the teen remarks listed earlier, the following might work: "What happened when you two

talked about this?" "What are your thoughts about dealing with this situation?"

4. Ask for details to clarify a problem or situation if more information seems important for the discussion and your child is not offering this. For example: "What was going on when the kids started calling you these names?" "What are the things that you would like to do on your dates that Dylan makes fun of?"

5. To share your thoughts or feelings, speak straightforwardly for yourself with "I" statements. "I'm glad you brought this up." "I mention this because I am worried." "I want to share with you what I know about this topic." "I am concerned because I feel, from what you just said, that you don't want me to meet your boyfriend." "I want to talk to you about this even if it is a little awkward for both of us."

6. Don't mind-read and tell your child what he or she is thinking or feeling. Avoid starting statements with "you." "You" statements often end up as the five P's—for example, "You just want to have your own way on this." Explore, through listening and open-ended questions, for what your child is actually thinking, feeling, and wanting. When you get a response, check out your impressions to be sure you are both on the same wavelength.

7. Selectively share personal information about yourself, about your own youth, about your knowledge level, about how you arrive at decisions, and the like, if you think a personal disclosure is appropriate for this topic and will benefit your child. Make sure that your child understands that your sharing is to help him or her better understand the sexual matter at hand. For example, "It took me a long time to learn that women are entitled to enjoy sexual pleasure." "I got into several relationships that weren't good for me, but I didn't have the maturity to get out of them when I should have." "I had a girlfriend who tried to kill herself when her boyfriend broke up with her."

8. Be prepared to appropriately assert your privacy if your child should press for details that you think are out of bounds. "What I

just told you about was my choice to share. But the details of my personal life are private."

9. Include remarks that show care, support, and positive valuing of your child's part in the discussion. "I see you putting a lot of thought into making this decision." "I'm glad you spoke your opinions even if they disagreed with mine." "I think your understanding of sex and our family's values will help you have a good life."

10. Find ways to put a positive frame or "spin" on the sexual topic or problem under discussion and especially to capture the fact that sexuality is a normal and rich dimension of life. This has to flow from your honest belief. This framing could include, for example, comments like these: "The way that you're struggling with this problem shows responsibility." "There's a lot to enjoy about your sexuality along with the difficulties and risks." "Getting to know about your own body and sexual sensations is normal." "Your excitement about this boy is great and part of growing up and beginning to learn about love." "You can't be prepared for everything that happens in sex and love, but people learn from mistakes how to have a happy life."

Guidelines for Conveying Sexual Information

Throughout this book, I have offered numerous suggestions to help you effectively provide sexual information to your child. These and other guidelines bear repeating here. Real conversations will call for you to blend both sexual information and moral guidance in ways that keep the conversation alive. First, we will look at guidelines for conveying information and then consider guidelines for incorporating moral and ethical issues.

1. Clarify what sexual information the discussion calls for. Do this by listening and exploring the situation or question and by asking for your child's understanding of the sexual matter.

2. In general, discuss needed sexual information before moving into moral and ethical values, beliefs, and guidelines.

3. If your child seems lacking in information, present and explain the needed facts. If he or she mentions sexual misinformation or myths, respectfully offer additional information to correct these.

4. Acknowledge when you need more information to clarify a sexual matter and mention your willingness to obtain it.

5. It is often helpful to give information about sexual attitudes, behaviors, risks, and beliefs in terms of "people in general," "what we know about kids," and so on.

6. When the focus is on sexual facts and the need for full information, go into sufficient detail to make the information meaningful and useful. For example, explain exactly what to expect in a gynecological exam, or the details of menstruation and wet dreams, or the mechanics of using a condom, or the communication skills needed to say no to sex.

7. Offer your child more books or specialized books on the subject or express your willingness to look further at details that are in your own or your teenager's books on sexuality.

Guidelines for Conveying Moral and Ethical Values and Beliefs

You should not shy away from having a give-and-take discussion with teenagers about moral beliefs. Even if your teen doesn't initially bring up his or her personal beliefs or those of others who might disagree with your views, you can be sure that he or she has come across many different viewpoints about sexuality and sexual conduct. As mentioned before, if you have worked to clarify your moral and ethical beliefs, you can feel confident in getting your values out in the open. Otherwise, your child may automatically adopt the sexual values of friends and the media. The basic communication skills presented earlier will help you carry out the following guidelines for *blending* moral and ethical guidance with sexual information.

1. Unless a sexual discussion begins with your moral or ethical beliefs about sexuality, don't start a conversation with your views.

Although your son or daughter might know your values, your stating these right from the beginning can discourage a teenager from bringing up possible opposing values or beliefs for discussion.

2. Give openings or lead-ins to encourage your child to mention moral and ethical beliefs that others might hold or those that are different from the family's values.

3. Be selective about which moral and ethical values you bring up, making sure that they fit the situation.

4. Present your values in a way that matches the maturity level of the child. With a young teen, you might strongly endorse or give a strict interpretation of certain values. With an older teen, you might allow more flexibility in your talk about values and morality, if this shift fits your beliefs. Distinguish between rules of conduct for adults, who can assume responsibility for all outcomes, and rules for young people, who are not in a position to take on adult obligations.

5. When you relate your beliefs, values, and advice to your child, put these in the form of "I" or "we" statements that include your hopes, dreams, and expectations for your child: "I hope that you will give yourself time to learn the difference between infatuation and love." "I expect that you will treat your girlfriend with respect and care for her as a person." "We expect that you will not engage in sexual intercourse while you're a teenager." "We expect you to be 100 percent responsible and protect yourself and your partner if you engage in intimate sexual activity."

6. Make it a point to convey sexual values that you believe in, not simply those that you think you *should* provide to your child.

7. Make it a point to include among your values the positive dimensions of sexuality and its relationship to human well-being and happiness.

The communication skills that enable you to have good sex talks with teenagers are demanding. Sensitive communication is necessary because young people in the hot zone of adolescence are as complicated as adults, maybe more so. With their new emotions and sexual urges, greater freedom, and a life outside the family home, young people want more privacy for their lives. You need to continue to treat sexual matters as a normal subject of family discussion. At the same time, you need to respect the young person's more personal response to this topic and realize that most of your sexual discussions will likely be one-on-one rather than open family discussions.

Practice Makes Perfect

A few training exercises will help you try your hand with the important communication skills discussed in this chapter. To begin practice, get a clean pad of paper and a pen. Several vignettes here suggest a sexual matter that might come up in the course of a discussion with a teenager. Whether you have a child this age or not, complete the practice and invite your partner to participate too. First, scan the vignettes, then follow the directions that explain how to practice.

1. Your sixteen-year-old son, after talking with you about a homework assignment, hangs around making small talk and mentions, "This kid I know at school. He told me that he's been stealing women's underwear from the mall, and wearing it at night, and sometimes at school. Is that weird or what?"

2. Your fourteen-year-old daughter, while watching a television movie with you, brings up the following question that doesn't seem to have anything to do with the movie: "I know what the books say about homosexuals, but what's with lesbians? Do they just hate men and that's why they would turn to a woman for love?"

3. You have had a few exchanges with your sixteen-year-old daughter about how the media present unrealistic portrayals about love. One evening, while watching television with you, she challenges you with this remark: "If marriage and sex aren't like the way they show them in the movies, what's the point of getting married?

Isn't passionate love what everyone wants? Marriage must be a big disappointment."

4. You come home from work early one afternoon and find your thirteen-year-old son watching the *Jerry Springer Show*, which is off-limits according to family rules. He responds, "I don't see anything wrong with this show. All my friends watch it, and we just think it's funny. I don't see why you think it's bad."

5. While driving with your seventeen-year-old daughter after a shopping trip together, she seems to be in a talkative mood and asks, "What is the big deal about being a virgin anyway? A lot of kids who say they're virgins do 'everything but' and I do mean everything. Isn't that hypocritical?"

For each vignette, you will practice a response based on all of the ten communication skills explained earlier. Be sure to *write* your responses as the directions state, rather than just think about them. Follow these steps, starting with the first vignette.

1. Rate your comfort level for the vignette, using this rating scale: 1 = can handle; 2 = worry about this one; 3 = wish to avoid; 4 = unprepared and unwilling. The rating will suggest your readiness for the topic with regard to emotions and knowledge.

2. Read the vignette again, and then go back to the beginning of the section titled "Important Communication Skills." Taking one skill at a time, formulate a response that demonstrates each of the skills in this section. Because skill 1 is about listening, begin with skill 2, which calls for a response that reflects the thought or feeling behind the teen's question. For example, in the first vignette, you might say, "You seem pretty shocked by what the kid told you." Write your response, and then speak it aloud. Then go on and formulate a response using skill 3 with the same vignette and write your response. Consider all the skills through skill 10, but if one does not seem applicable for the situation, skip that one and go on to the next. Remember to write *and speak* your responses.

3. Continue using the same vignette and review the section titled "Guidelines for Conveying Sexual Information." Think about how the skills you just practiced (look at your written responses) would help you carry out these guidelines in a conversation about the topic in the vignette. For example, you might think, "I can see that it is important to ask for clarification, without interrogating, about why the friend might have told about the underwear."

4. Continue using the same vignette and review the section titled "Guidelines for Conveying Moral and Ethical Values and Beliefs." Think about how the skills you just practiced (look at your written responses) would help you carry out these guidelines in a conversation about the topic in the vignette. For example, you might think, "I can see how all the skills could keep me from jumping in immediately with a premature moral judgment about a boy who wears female underwear, which could quickly end my conversation with my son."

5. Once you have finished practicing with the first vignette, follow these same steps for the remaining ones.

When the topic of sex education comes up, most adults automatically think of adolescents and lament, mentally if not verbally, about all the sexual problems of youth. This mind-set stereotypes all teens and essentially reduces them to genitals and ignores their hearts, minds, and souls. Because of this tendency, we need reminders to learn and use effective communication with our teenagers.

This very conscious approach might not be so necessary if we could see youngsters as the whole persons that they are. Their lives, like those of adults, consist of balancing daily responsibilities with the task of growing up. They wonder what school and jobs will have to do with their future. They worry about how to present themselves, whether others will like them, and if they will be good enough. They look for fun, challenges, and the thrill and excitement of having a special romantic partner. At the same time, they struggle to find the right balance between attempting to meet the expectations of their families or friends and finding their own way. For all they are and do, our adolescents deserve our continued love, nurturance, and respect. With the next stage, young adulthood, comes the sense that they are at last their own person and thus ready to intensify the search for a special mate.

Epilogue

The promise that I made at the beginning of this book can become a reality. You can overcome the personal hang-ups that keep you from giving your child the kind of sex and moral education that you believe in. I know the ideas and exercises here will work because I have seen parents use and benefit from them.

During the final months of writing this book, a colleague and I offered several group educational workshops for mothers who were interested in becoming active and influential in their child's sex education. (Only mothers were in these first experimental programs because we knew that quickly recruiting mothers would be easier than getting both mothers and fathers to participate.) In the beginning, they were, like most parents, committed to helping their child with the difficult topic of sex, but tentative, embarrassed, and uncertain about how to take on this parental duty that no one ever talks about.

The mothers who attended held different views about the topic of sex education and the role of parents. A few had taken small steps toward giving their child sexual information, whereas others had done nothing and worried about missed opportunities. They also differed somewhat in regard to their moral and ethical values and their general comfort with sexual topics. Regardless, every mother wanted to do her best to foster her child's healthy sexual development and was ready and willing to learn.

These parents discovered immediately that we *can* talk about sex in a thoughtful way—in spite of the cultural message telling us not to. At times we couldn't get them to stop talking! They willingly shared stories about their own lives. They were fascinated by sexual information that was new to them. They appreciated learning from each other. And they often tapped into their own wisdom and became more willing to share that with their child.

The mothers in the groups took other steps that I believe this book can help you take as well. They moved into the action phase of putting their learning into practice—almost immediately for some. Their experience in the group took them beyond the benefits of private learning, sharing with other women, support, and fun with the subject matter. One mother e-mailed me this reaction: "On the way home I stopped at the bookstore and purchased two books, . . . *The Big Secret* and *It's a Girl Thing.* We used the first book after dinner that night to introduce the topic of where and how babies are created and sexuality. This was a great opening discussion and our four- and seven-year old sons had very perceptive questions. . . . The latter book . . . with my daughter, who is nine . . . has opened the door to more conversations about puberty."

The mother of a nine-year-old boy wrote, "The information was great; however, I may not remember it all for when I'll need it. The good thing is that I am aware of more resources now than I was before I participated in the group." Within several months she wrote again saying that she had had a wonderful introductory talk with her son about sex and that she was surprised that it had gone so well and her son had been so receptive: "We discussed everything from wet dreams to menstruation to actual intercourse! He was very comfortable as was I about this, and we both had fun with it."

My firsthand experience with mothers who valued and used the approach in this book is gratifying. It convinced me that we have to do more than offer simple platitudes—"sex education belongs in the family" and the like. Our young people do face a crisis that threatens their sexual health, and parents are in the best position to prepare them with both accurate sexual information and a solid grounding in character and moral development. Parents will take on this responsibility, but they often need a step-by-step guide for how to act on their good intentions.

By reading and interacting with this book, you can be a part of making family-based sex education a reality. But it doesn't happen magically or all at once. It's necessary for mothers and fathers to work together, identify and overcome their hang-ups, clarify moral values, update their knowledge of sexuality, and then start the life-long process of sharing information and moral guidance with their child.

I also invite you to take the message beyond your own family. Talk to others about children's need for sex education: to your spouse or partner, relatives, friends, neighbors. Bring up the subject in public discussions, such as in religious groups, parent-teacher association meetings, and community service organizations. One parent at time, one family at a time, one organization at a time—we can make a difference not only in the sexual health of our own child but also for the coming generation and for society in general.

Resources

Adult and Couple Sexuality and Relationship Concerns

Bass, Ellen, and Laura Davis. *The Courage to Heal: A Guide for Women Survivors of Child Sexual Abuse*. New York: HarperCollins, 1988.

Castleman, Michael. *Sexual Solutions: A Guide for Men and the Women Who Love Them*. New York: Simon & Schuster, 1983.

DeVillers, Linda. *Love Skills: More Fun Than You've Ever Had with Sex, Intimacy, and Communication*. San Luis Obispo, Calif.: Impact, 1997.

Engel, Bernard F. *Raising Your Self-Esteem: How to Feel Better About Your Sexuality and Yourself*. New York: Ballantine, 1995.

Heiman, Julia, and Joseph Lo Piccolo. *Becoming Orgasmic: A Sexual and Personal Growth Program for Women*. New York: Fireside, 1988.

Louden, James K. *The Couple's Comfort Book: A Creative Guide for Renewing Passion, Pleasure, and Commitment*. San Francisco: Harper San Francisco, 1994.

Maltz, Wendy. *The Sexual Healing Journey*. New York: HarperCollins, 1991.

McCarthy, Barry. *Male Sexual Awareness: Increasing Sexual Satisfaction*. New York: Carroll & Graf, 1988.

McCarthy, Barry, and Elizabeth McCarthy. *Female Sexual Awareness and Sexual Fulfillment*. New York: Carroll & Graf, 1989.

Pittman, Frank S., III. *Man Enough: Fathers, Sons, and the Search for Masculinity*. New York: Putnam, 1993.

Renshaw, Domeena. *Seven Weeks to Better Sex*. New York: Dell, 1995.

Schaefer, Charles E., and Theresa Foy DiGeronimo. *How to Talk to Your Kids About Really Important Things*. San Francisco: Jossey-Bass, 1994.

Schaefer, Charles E., and Theresa Foy DiGeronimo. *How to Talk to Your Teens About Really Important Things*. San Francisco: Jossey-Bass, 1999.

Wallerstein, Judith S., and Sandra Blakeslee. *The Good Marriage: How and Why Love Lasts*. Boston: Houghton Mifflin, 1995.

Zilbergeld, Bernie. *The New Male Sexuality*. New York: Bantam Books, 1992.

Sex Education Resources

For Parents

Books

Acker, Loren E., Brian C. Goldwater, and William H. Dyson. *AIDS-Proofing Your Kids: A Step-by-Step Guide*. Hillsboro, Oreg.: Beyond Words, 1992.

Blankenhorn, David. *Fatherless America: Confronting Our Most Urgent Social Problem*. New York: Basic Books, 1995.

Borhek, M. V. *Coming Out to Parents: A Two-Way Survival Guide for Lesbians and Gay Men and Their Parents*. New York: Pilgrim, 1983.

Cassell, Carol. *Straight from the Heart: How to Talk to Your Teenagers About Love and Sex*. New York: Simon & Schuster, 1987.

De Freitas, Chrystal. *Keys to Your Child's Healthy Sexuality*. Hauppage, N.Y.: Barron's, 1998.

Eagle, Carol J., and Carol Coleman. *All That She Can Be*. New York: Simon & Schuster, 1993.

Gale, John. *A Parent's Guide to Teenage Sexuality*. New York: Henry Holt, 1989.

Gordon, Sol, and Judith Gordon. *Raising a Child Responsibly in a Sexually Permissive World*. Holbrook, Mass.: Adams Media, 2000.

Madaras, Lynda. *Lynda Madaras Talks to Teens About AIDS: An Essential Guide for Parents, Teachers, and Young People*. New York: Newmarket Press, 1988.

McNaught, Brian. *Now That I'm Out, What Do I Do?* New York: Bedford/St. Martin's, 1998.

McNaught, Brian. *On Being Gay*. New York: Bedford/St. Martin's, 1988.

Planned Parenthood. *Talking About Sex: A Guide for Families*. New York: Planned Parenthood Federation of America, 1996. Includes video.

Tally, Scott. *Talking with Your Kids About the Birds and the Bees*. Ventura, Calif.: Gospel Light, 1990.

Vaughan, Peggy, and James Vaughan. *Sex Education: For Parents Only*. Copyright © 1996. Available: http://www.oeg.net/vaughan/sex.html

Walker, Richard. *The Family Guide to Sex and Relationships*. Old Tappan, N.J.: Macmillan, 1996.

Warren, Andrea, and Jay Wiedenkeller. *Everybody's Doing It*. New York: Penguin, 1993.

Religious Sources

Several sources in these lists of readings are from publishing companies affili-
ated with a religious perspective. For specific denominational information, the
following bibliographies may be useful: *Current Religious Perspectives on Sexuality*
and *Sexuality Education Resources for Religious Denominations*. These may be purchased from SIECUS, 130 West Forty-Second Street, Suite 350, New York, NY
10036.

Eyre, Linda, and Richard Eyre. *How to Talk to Your Child About Sex*. New York:
Bedford/St. Martin's, 1998. This book provides a traditional approach to sex
education based on abstinence until marriage.

Our Whole Lives (OWL). Faith-based sexuality education program. Developed
jointly by the United Church of Christ (ucc.org) and the Unitarian Universalist
Association (uua.org).

Pamphlets and Videotapes Available from Planned Parenthood

Most Planned Parenthood agencies have books and other resources available
for loan. Individual copies of pamphlets are usually free, such as the following:
*A Man's Guide to Sexuality; Feeling Good About Growing Up; Teensex? It's Okay
to Say: No Way!; Human Sexuality: What Children Should Know and When They
Should Know It; Kids and AIDS: A Guide for Parents; How to Talk with Your Child
About Sexuality: A Parent's Guide;* and *How to Talk with Your Teen About the Facts
of Life*.

Most Planned Parenthood agencies also offer educational videotapes to borrow
for a small fee. Many of these are designed for parents and children to watch
together. Titles will likely vary with different Planned Parenthood locations.
The following are some typical titles: *Talking About Sex: A Guide for Families; A
Million Teenagers* (for fourteen- to eighteen-year-olds); *What Kids Want to Know
About Sex and Growing Up* (for eight- to twelve-year-olds); *Can We Talk? Helping
Families Talk About Self-Esteem, Sex, and Peer Pressure; Sex: A Topic of Conversa-
tion with Dr. Sol Gordon: For Parents of Small Children; Bellybuttons Are Navels*.

Selected Videotapes for Purchase

AIDS Awareness for Teens
Teacher's Video Company
P.O. Box ASHA-4455
Scottsdale, AZ 85261
(800) 262-8837

Raising Sexually Healthy Children
Magna Systems, Inc.
95 West County Line Road
Barrington, IL 60010
(800) 203-7060; fax order (815) 459-4280
E-mail: magnasys@ix.netcom.com

Sex and Other Matters of Life and Death (for parents)
The Cinema Guild, Inc.
1697 Broadway, Suite 506
New York, NY 10019
(212) 246-5522; (800) 723-5522
E-mail: TheCinemaG@aol.com

Sex and Other Matters of Life and Death (for students/classroom use)
AGC Educational Media
1560 Sherman Avenue, Suite 100
Evanston, IL 60201
(847) 328-6700; (800) 323-9084
E-mail: agcmedia@starnetinc.com

Sexuality in a Culture of Confusion
Media Education Foundation
26 Center Street
Northampton, MA 01060
(800) 897-0089
E-mail: mediaed@mediaed.org

For Toddlers and Young Children

Brown, Laurie. *What's the Big Secret?* New York: Little, Brown, 1997.
Jeffs, Stephanie, and Jane Coulson. *The Miracle of Life*. Nashville, Tenn.: Abingdon Press, 1998.
Mantegazza, Giovanna. *Look How a Baby Grows,* trans. Alexandra E. Fischer; ill. Anna Curti. New York: Grosset & Dunlap, 1995.
Mayle, Peter. *"Where Did I Come From?" The Facts of Life Without Any Nonsense and with Illustrations*. Secaucus, N.J.: Carol, 1999. (Also available in an African American edition)
Smith, Alistair. *How Are Babies Made?* Tulsa, Okla.: EDC, 1998.

For Elementary School Age Children

Aho, Jennifer, and John W. Petras. *Learning About Sex.* New York: Henry Holt, 1995.

Gardner-Loulan, JoAnn, and Bonnie Lopez. *Period.* (Rev. ed.) Volcano, Calif.: Volcano Press, 1991.

Gitchel, Sam, and Lorri Foster. *Let's Talk About . . . S-E-X.* Fresno: Planned Parenthood of Central California, 1995.

Harris, Robie H. *It's Perfectly Normal.* Cambridge, Mass.: Candlewick Press, 1994.

Jukes, Mavis. *Growing Up: It's a Girl Thing.* New York: Random House/Knopf, 1998.

Jukes, Mavis. *It's a Girl Thing: How to Stay Healthy, Safe, and in Charge.* New York: Random House/Knopf, 1997.

Marsh, Carole. *Sex Stuff for Kids Seven to Seventeen.* Atlanta: Gallopade, 1994.

Thomson, Ruth. *Have You Started Yet?* New York: Price, Stern, Sloan, 1995.

Westheimer, Ruth. *Dr. Ruth Talks to Kids: Where You Came From, How Your Body Changes, and What Sex Is All About.* New York: Simon & Schuster, 1993.

For Adolescents

Abner, Allison, and Linda Villarosa. *Finding Our Way: The Teen Girls' Survival Guide.* New York: HarperCollins, 1995.

Akagi, Cynthia. *Dear Larissa: Sexuality Education for Girls Eleven to Seventeen.* Littleton, Colo.: Gylantic, 1994.

Bell, Ruth. *Changing Bodies, Changing Lives.* (3rd ed.) New York: Random House, 1998.

Bouris, Karen. *The First Time.* Berkeley, Calif.: Conari Press, 1995.

Bull, David. *Cool and Celibate? Sex or No Sex?* Bodon, Mass.: Element Books, 1998.

Gurian, Michael. *From Boys to Men: All About Adolescence and You.* New York: Price, Stern, Sloan, 1999.

Gurian, Michael. *Understanding Guys: A Guide for Teenage Girls.* New York: Price, Stern, Sloan, 1999.

Huron, Ann. *Two Teenagers in Twenty: Writings by Gay and Lesbian Youth.* Boston: Alyson, 1994.

Johnson, Eric. *Love and Sex in Plain Language.* New York: HarperCollins, 1985.

Lester, Teri. *Healthy Love: A Step-by-Step Method for Practicing Abstinence.* Overland Park, Kans.: RUC, 1994.

Madaras, Lynda. *Lynda Madaras Talks to Teens About AIDS: An Essential Guide for Parents, Teachers, and Young People.* New York: Newmarket Press, 1988.

Madaras, Lynda. *The "What's Happening to My Body?" Book for Boys.* New York: Newmarket Press, 1988.

Madaras, Lynda. The "What's Happening to My Body?" Book for Girls. New York: Newmarket Press, 1988.

Marsh, Carole. Sex Stuff for Kids Seven to Seventeen. Atlanta: Gallopade, 1994.

McCoy, Kathy, and Charles Wibbelsman. The New Teenage Body Book. New York: Berkley, 1992.

Nonkin, Lesley Jane. I Wish My Parents Understood. New York: Penguin, 1985.

Parrot, Andrea. Coping with Date Rape and Acquaintance Rape. New York: Rosen, 1988.

Pogany, Susan B. Sex Smart: 501 Reasons to Hold Off on Sex. Minneapolis, Minn.: Fairview Press, 1998.

Rench, Janice E. Understanding Sexual Identity: A Book for Gay Teens and Their Friends. Minneapolis, Minn.: Lerner, 1990.

Scott, Sharon. How to Say No and Keep Your Friends. Amherst, Mass.: Human Resource Development Press, 1986.

Short, Ray E. Sex, Love, or Infatuation: How Can I Really Know? Minneapolis, Minn.: Augsburg Fortress, 1990.

Smith, Manuel J. Yes, I Can Say No. New York: Arbor House, 1986.

Stoppard, Miriam. Sex Ed: Growing Up, Relationships, and Sex. New York: D.K., 1997.

Westheimer, Ruth, and Nathan Kravatz. First Love: A Young People's Guide to Sexual Information. New York: Warner Books, 1985.

Weston, Carol. Girltalk: All the Stuff Your Sister Never Told You. New York: HarperCollins, 1985.

Woods, Samuel G. Everything You Need to Know About STD: Sexually Transmitted Disease. New York: Rosen, 1990.

Organizations and Internet Information Sources

American Association for Marriage and Family Therapy
1133 Fifteenth Street, NW, Suite 300
Washington, DC 20005
(202) 452-0109; fax: (202) 223-2329
http://www.aamft.org

American Association of Sex Educators, Counselors and Therapists (AASECT)
P.O. Box 5488
Richmond, VA 23220
(804) 644-3288; fax (804) 644-3290
E-mail: aasect@mediaone.net

American Association on Mental Retardation
444 North Capitol Street, NW, Suite 846
Washington, DC 20001
(800) 424-3688

Colage: Children of Lesbians and Gays Everywhere
2300 Market Street, Box 165
San Francisco, CA 94114
(415) 861-KIDS
E-mail: KIDSOFGAYS@aol.com

Gay and Lesbian Parents Coalition International (GLPCI)
P.O. Box 50360
Washington, DC 20091
(202) 583-8029
E-mail: glpcinat@ix.netcom.com

GIRLS, INC
Resource Center
441 West Michigan Street
Indianapolis, IN 46202
(800) 374-4475

GIRL POWER!
Department of Health and Human Services
National Clearinghouse for Alcohol and Drug Information (NCADI)
(800) 729-6686; TDD: (800) 487-4889
http://www.health.org/gpower

Go Ask Alice
(Columbia University)
http://www.goaskalice.columbia.edu

Mothers' Voices
165 W. Forty-Sixth Street, Suite 701
New York, NY 10036
(212) 730-2777; (888) MVOICES; fax: (212) 730-4378
http://www.mvoices.org

National Campaign to Prevent Teen Pregnancy
1776 Massachusetts Avenue, NW, Suite 200
Washington, DC 20036
(202) 857-8655; fax: (202) 331-7735
http://www.teenpregnancy.org

National Gay and Lesbian Task Force
2320 Seventeenth Street, NW
Washington, DC 20009
(202) 332-6483

Network for Family Life Education
(Rutgers University)
E-mail: sxetc@rci.rutgers.edu

Parents and Friends of Lesbians and Gays (P-FLAG)
1101 Fourteenth Street, NW, Suite 1030
Washington, DC 20005
(202) 638-4200; fax: (202) 638-0243
E-mail: INFO@PFLAG.ORG

Planned Parenthood Federation of America
810 Seventh Avenue
New York, NY 10019
(800) 669-0156; fax: (212) 261-4352
http://www.ppfa.org

Religious Coalition for Reproductive Choice
1025 Vermont Avenue, NW, Suite 1130
Washington, DC 20005
(202) 628-7700; fax: (202) 628-7716
E-mail: info@rerc.org
http://www.rcrc.org

Sexuality and Disability Training Center
University Hospital
75 East Newton Street
Boston, MA 02118
(617) 638-7358

Sexuality and Information Council of the United States (SIECUS)
Publications Department
130 West Forty-Second Street, Suite 350
New York, NY 10036
(212) 819-9770; fax: (212) 819-9776
http://www.siecus.org

Society for the Scientific Study of Sex
P.O. Box 416
Allentown, PA 18105
(610) 530-2483

Talking with Kids About Tough Issues
http://www.talkingwithkids.org

Teenwire
http://www.teenwire.com

Notes

Preface

1. *Tallahassee Democrat*, July 17–20, 1996.

Introduction

1. For research findings on the negative effects of the media, see Edward Donnerstein, "The Media as Sex Educator," *Contemporary Sexuality*, 1999, *33*(3), 1, 2, 8.

2. For discussion of the impact of the Internet and media on children, see Al Cooper, "The Internet and Sexuality: Into the Next Millennium," *Journal of Sex Education and Therapy*, 1997, *22*(1), 5–6.

3. National Association of Missing and Exploited Children, 2000, http://www.missingkids.org.

4. The quotation on pop culture appeared in Donnerstein, "The Media as Sex Educator," p. 2.

5. Ron Taffel, "The Second Family," *Family Therapy Networker*, 1996, *20*(3), 36–45.

6. The impact of youth culture is discussed in Robert E. Fullilove, Warren Barksdale, and Mindy Thompson Fullilove, "Teens Talk Sex: Can We Talk Back?" in Janice M. Irvine (ed.), *Sexual Culture and the Construction of Adolescent Identities* (Philadelphia: Temple University Press, 1994), p. 321.

7. The survey on boys' and girls' concerns appeared in Bridget Murray, "Survey Reveals Concerns of Today's Girls," *American Psychological Association Monitor*, 1998, *12*(10), 12.

8. Parents' underestimation of teens' sexual activity is reported in James Jaccard and Patricia J. Dittus, *Parent-Teen Communication: Toward the Prevention of Unintended Pregnancies* (New York: Springer-Verlag, 1991).

9. The news reports cited are from the *Omaha World Herald*, May 19, 2000, pp. 1, 12; June 2, 2000, p. 13; Jan. 9, 2001, p. 9.

10. The teen focus group discussions of sex were reported in Joe Fay and Jay M. Yanoff, "What Are Teens Telling Us About Sexual Health? Results of the Second Annual Youth Conference of the Pennsylvania Coalition to Prevent Teen Pregnancy," *Journal of Sex Education and Therapy*, 2000, 25(2–3), 169–177.

11. Findings on parents' views on masturbation appeared in Nathaniel McConaghy, *Sexual Behavior: Problems and Management* (New York: Plenum Press, 1993).

12. Incongruency between parents' and teens' reports of sexual talks was reported in James Jaccard, Patricia J. Dittus, and Vivian V. Gordon, "Parent-Adolescent Congruency in Reports of Adolescent Sexual Behavior and in Communication About Sexual Behavior," *Child Development*, 1998, 69, 247–261.

13. The lack of parent involvement in the AIDS education program was reported in *Sex Weekly*, 1996, (Sample issue, n.d.), p. 19.

14. Teens' views on parents' sex education was reported in Kay E. Mueller and William G. Powers, "Parent-Child Sexual Discussion: Perceived Communication Style and Subsequent Behavior," *Adolescence*, 1990, 25, 469–482. This article extensively reviews research over the past twenty years that reports teens' perceptions of the role of parents in their sex education.

15. Parents' wishes for schools to teach more sexual topics appeared in Todd Melby, "Sex Ed Study: Big Gap Between Parental Desires and Classroom Realities," *Contemporary Sexuality*, 2000, 34(12), 1, 4–5. This review is based on "Sex in America: A View from Inside the Nation's Classrooms," a study by the Henry J. Kaiser Family Foundation (KFF). A summary report , including the questionnaire and major findings, is available at http://www.kff.org or by calling KFF at (800) 656-4533. If calling, ask for no. 3048.

16. The quotation about Monica Lewinsky is from Mona Charen, Creators Syndicate, Washington, D.C., Mar. 5, 1999.

17. For the report of parents' wishes for school sex education programs, see Melby, "Sex Ed Study."

18. The failure of public school sex education programs to uphold democratic ideals is discussed in John P. Elia, "Democratic Sexuality Education: A Departure from Sexual Ideologies and Traditional Schooling," *Journal of Sex Education and Therapy*, 2000, 25, 122–129. The original source is Alexander McKay, *Sexual Ideology and Schooling: Toward a Democratic Sexuality Education* (New York: State University of New York Press, 1999).

19. For a review of federally supported abstinence-based sex education, see Michael Young and Eva S. Goldfarb, "The Problematic (a)–(h) in

Abstinence Education," *Journal of Sex Education and Therapy*, 2000, 25(2–3), 156–160.

20. The components of abstinence-based education from the Welfare Reform Act of 1996, P.L. 104-193, Title V, Sec. 510, are quoted from Young and Goldfarb, "The Problematic (a)–(h)," p. 157.

21. Recent historical accounts of the sexual revolution include David Allyn, *Make Love, Not War: The Sexual Revolution—an Unfettered History* (Boston: Little, Brown, 2000); Beth Bailey, *Sex in the Heartland* (Cambridge, Mass.: Harvard University Press, 1999); and John Heidenry, *What Wild Ecstasy: The Rise and Fall of the Sexual Revolution* (New York: Simon & Schuster, 1999).

22. The quotation about boomers' moral contradictions is from Allyn, *Make Love, Not War*, p. 294.

23. The quotation about fathers' views on abstinence is from Georgia Witkin, Ph.D., *Beyond the News*, Fox News Channel, Nov. 21, 1999.

1. Taking a Personal Inventory for Moms

1. Many sources document the negative slurs directed toward girls' sexuality. See, for example, Sue Lees, *Sugar and Spice: Sexuality and Adolescent Girls* (New York: Penguin, 1993), and Peggy Orenstein, *School Girls: Young Women, Self-Esteem, and the Confidence Gap* (New York: Anchor Books, 1994).

2. The Ann Landers survey was discussed in Kevin Klose, "Ann Landers' Tide of Discontent: In Sex Survey 60,000 Women Tell Columnist They'd Rather Be Hugged," *Washington Post*, Jan. 15, 1981, p. C1.

3. This research reflects similar findings from many studies of vast differences in boys' and girls' reports of pleasure from intercourse. The study cited is reported in Jane D. Woody, Robin Russel, Henry J. D'Souza, and Jennifer Woody, "Adolescent Non-Coital Sexual Activity: Comparisons of Virgins and Non-Virgins," *Journal of Sex Education and Therapy*, 2000, 25, 261–268.

4. Kathy Dobie, "Hellbent on Redemption," *Mother Jones*, Jan.-Feb. 1995, p. 50.

5. For an analysis of the prevalence of sexual dysfunction in the general population, see Edward O. Lauman, Anthony Paik, and Raymond C. Rosen, "Sexual Dysfunction in the United States: Prevalence and Predictors," *Journal of the American Medical Association*, 1999, 281, 537–544.

6. Research on interaction that predicts marital stability appeared in John Gottman, "Why Marriages Fail," *Family Therapy Networker*, May–June 1994, 18, 41–48.

2. Taking a Personal Inventory for Dads

1. For a discussion of the centerfold syndrome and nonrelational sex, see Ronald F. Levant and Gary R. Brooks, *Men and Sex* (New York: Wiley, 1995), p. 31.
2. Boys' social programming and the "boy code" are discussed in William Pollack, *Real Boys: Rescuing Our Sons from the Myths of Boyhood* (New York: Random House, 1998).
3. For a current detailed report on both men's and women's sexual attitudes and behaviors, see Robert T. Michael, John H. Gagnon, Edward O. Lauman, and Gina Kolata, *Sex in America: A Definitive Survey* (New York: Little, Brown, 1994); Levant and Brooks, *Men and Sex*.
4. For reports on adolescents' sexual knowledge and early sexual activities, see Kay E. Mueller and William G. Powers, "Parent-Child Sexual Discussion: Perceived Communicator Style and Subsequent Behavior," *Adolescence*, 1990, 25(98), 469–482; Floyd M. Martinson, *The Sexual Life of Children* (Westport, Conn.: Bergin & Garvey, 1994).
5. For an analysis of the prevalence of sexual dysfunction in the general population, see Lauman, Paik, and Rosen, "Sexual Dysfunction in the United States."
6. Research on interaction that predicts marital stability appeared in Gottman, "Why Marriages Fail."
7. Research on influences on youths' sexual decisions appeared in Jane D. Woody, Robin Russel, and Henry J. D'Souza, "Parental Influence on Adolescent Sexual Decisions: The Perspective of Young Adults," unpublished manuscript, 2001.
8. This sex education curriculum for boys is excellent. You may want to work toward getting this program in your community. For information, see Family Life Council of Greater Greensboro, *Wise Guys: Male Responsibility Curriculum* (Greensboro, N.C.: Family Life Council of Greater Greensboro, 1998).

3. Working Together as a Team

1. Among the most important studies that examine the association between youths' high-risk sexual behavior and parent and family factors are Deborah Holtzman and Richard Rubinson, "Parent and Peer Communication Effects on AIDS-Related Behavior Among U.S. High School Students," *Family Planning Perspectives*, 1995, 27, 235–240, 268; James Jaccard, Patricia J. Dittus, and Vivian V. Gordon, "Parent-Adolescent Congruency in Reports

of Adolescent Sexual Behavior and in Communication About Sexual Behavior," *Child Development*, 1998, *69*, 247–261; Frances Althaus, "Age at Which Young Men Initiate Intercourse Is Tied to Sex Education and Mother's Presence in the Home," *Family Planning Perspectives*, 1994, *26*, 142–143; Susan F. Newcomer and J. Richard Udry, "Mothers' Influence on the Sexual Behavior of Their Teenage Children," *Journal of Marriage and the Family*, 1984, *46*, 477–485; Michael Carrera, *The Language of Sex* (New York: Facts on File, 1992); Brent C. Miller, Maria C. Norton, Thom Curtis, E. Jeffrey Hill, Paul Schvaneveldt, and Margaret H. Young, "The Timing of Sexual Intercourse Among Adolescents: Family, Peer, and Other Antecedents," *Youth and Society*, 1997, *29*(1), 54–83; and Toon W. Taris, Gun R. Semin, and Inge A. Bok, "The Effect of Quality of Family Interaction and Intergenerational Transmission of Values on Sexual Permissiveness," *Journal of Genetic Psychology*, 1998, *159*, 237–250.

2. For more information about mentoring programs or special community initiatives on sex education, see Family Life Council, *Wise Guys*.

3. For a review of studies dealing with risks associated with early pubertal development, see Brent C. Miller, Maria C. Norton, Xitao Fan, and Cynthia R. Christopherson, "Pubertal Development, Parental Communication, and Sexual Values in Relation to Adolescent Sexual Behaviors," *Journal of Early Adolescence*, 1998, *18*, 27–52.

4. For a review of studies dealing with certain personality correlates of adolescent sexual behavior, see Miller and others, "The Timing of Sexual Intercourse." See also Les B. Whitbeck, Rand D. Conger, and Meei-Ying Kao, "The Influence of Parental Support, Depressed Affect, and Peers on the Sexual Behaviors of Adolescent Girls," *Journal of Family Issues*, 1993, *14*, 261–278, and Robert F. Valois, Sandra K. Kammermann, and J. Wanzer Drane, "Number of Sexual Intercourse Partners and Associated Risk Behaviors Among Public High School Adolescents," *Journal of Sex Education and Therapy*, 1997, *22*, 13–22. For a study exploring adult use of sexual Internet sites, see Alvin Cooper, Coralie Scherer, Sylvain C. Boies, and Barry Gordon, "Sexuality on the Internet: From Sexual Exploration to Pathological Expression," *Professional Psychology*, 1999, *30*, 154–164.

5. For details on gay and lesbian youth, see Paula K. Braverman and Victoria C. Strasburger, "Adolescent Sexual Activity," *Clinical Pediatrics*, 1993, *32*, 658–668; David W. Cramer and Arthur J. Roach, "Coming Out to Mom and Dad: A Study of Gay Males and Their Relationship with Their Parents," *Journal of Homosexuality*, 1988, *15*, 79–91; Robert Garofalo, R. Cameron Wolf, Shan Kessel, Judith Palfrey, and Robert H. DuRant, "The

Association Between Health-Risk Behaviors and Sexual Orientation Among a School-Based Sample of Adolescents," *Pediatrics*, 1998, *101*, 895–902; Scott S. Hersberger and Anthony R. D'Augelli, "The Impact of Victimization on the Mental Health and Suicidality of Lesbian, Gay, and Bisexual Youth," *Developmental Psychology*, 1995, *31*, 65–74; and Gabe Kruks, "Gay and Lesbian Homeless/Street Youth: Special Issues and Concerns," *Journal of Adolescent Health*, 1991, *12*, 515–518.

6. For further detail on gender identity disorder, see American Psychiatric Association, *Diagnostic and Statistical Manual of Mental Disorders* (4th ed.) (Washington, D.C.: American Psychiatric Association, 1994), and Susan J. Bradley and Kenneth J. Zucker, "Gender Identity Disorder and Psychosexual Problems in Children and Adolescents," *Canadian Journal of Psychiatry*, 1990, *35*, 477–486.

7. The cited prevalence rates for childhood sexual abuse are from David Finkelhor, Gina Hotaling, Irwin A. Lewis, and Christine Smith, "Sexual Abuse in a National Survey of Adult Men and Women: Prevalence, Characteristics, and Risk Factors," *Child Abuse and Neglect*, 1990, *14*, 19–28.

8. For recent studies on childhood sexual abuse and related sexual risks, see Clare E. Cosentino, Heino F. L. Meyer-Bahlburg, Judith L. Alpert, Sharon L. Weinberg, and Richard Gaines, "Sexual Behavior Problems and Psychopathology Symptoms in Sexually Abused Girls," *Journal of the American Academy of Child and Adolescent Psychiatry*, 1995, *34*, 1033–1042; David Skuse and others, "Risk Factors for Development of Sexually Abusive Behavior in Sexually Victimized Adolescent Boys: Cross-Sectional Study," *British Medical Journal*, 1998, *317*, 175–179; and Esther Deblinger and Anne Hope Heflin, *Treating Sexually Abused Children and Their Nonoffending Parents: A Cognitive Behavioral Approach* (Thousand Oaks, Calif.: Sage, 1996).

9. For further information on sexuality and childhood developmental disability, see Ann Craft, *Mental Handicap and Sexuality: Issues and Perspectives* (Turnbridge Wells, England: Costello, 1987); Rosalyn Kramer-Monat, *Sexuality and the Mentally Retarded* (San Diego, Calif.: College-Hill Press, 1982); Don C. Van Dyke, Dianne M. McBrien, and Andrea Sherbondy, "Issues of Sexuality in Down Syndrome," *Down Syndrome Research and Practice*, 1995, *3*, 65–69; and "Sexuality Education for Children and Adolescents with Developmental Disabilities," *Pediatrics*, 1996, *97*, 275–279.

10. The personal inventory showing characteristics of the sexually healthy adolescent is from Debra W. Haffner, "Facing Facts: Sexual Health for America's Adolescents," in *SIECUS Report*, Aug.-Sept. 1995; reprinted

with permission of SIECUS, 130 West Forty-Second Street, Suite 380, New York, NY 10036.

11. For further information on parents' divorce status and children's sexuality, see Frances Althaus, "Children from Disrupted Families Begin Having Sex, and Children, at Early Age," *Family Planning Perspectives*, 1997, *29*, 240–243, and Les B. Whitbeck, Ronald L. Simons, and Meei-Ying Kao, "The Effects of Divorced Mothers' Dating Behaviors and Sexual Attitudes on the Sexual Attitudes and Behaviors of Their Adolescent Children," *Journal of Marriage and the Family*, 1994, *56*, 615–621.

12. For further information on gay and lesbian parenting and child develop-ment, see Frederick W. Bozett (ed.), *Gay and Lesbian Parents* (New York: Praeger, 1987); April Martin, *The Lesbian and Gay Parenting Handbook* (New York: HarperCollins, 1993); Charlotte J. Patterson, "Lesbian Moth-ers, Gay Fathers, and Their Children," in Anthony R. D'Augelli and Charlotte J. Patterson (eds.), *Lesbian, Gay, and Bisexual Identities Across the Lifespan* (New York: Oxford University Press, 1995); Charlotte J. Patterson and Anthony R. D'Augelli (eds.), *Lesbian, Gay, and Bisexual Identities in Families: Psychological Perspectives* (New York: Oxford Univer-sity, Press, 1998); and Charlotte J. Patterson, "Lesbian and Gay Parent-hood," in Marc H. Bornstein (ed.), *Handbook of Parenting* (Mahwah, N.J.: Erlbaum, 1996).

4. Teaching Kids from One to Five

1. For a discussion of the emotional tasks of each childhood stage, see Erik H. Erikson, *Childhood and Society* (New York: Norton, 1950).

5. Teaching Kids from Six to Eleven

1. For the opinion that most children do not need sex education until puberty, see Barbara Dafoe Whitehead, "The Failure of Sex Education," *Atlantic*, Oct. 1994, pp. 55–80.

2. The viewpoint that children quickly learn not to ask about sex appears in Mary Calderone, "Adolescent Sexuality: Elements and Genesis," *Pediatrics*, 1985, *76*, 699–703.

3. For a discussion of children's emotional development, see Erik H. Erikson, *Childhood and Society*, 2nd ed., rev. (New York: Norton, 1964).

4. For a highly acclaimed young children's book that explains intercourse and pregnancy, see Peter Mayle, *"Where Did I Come From?"* (Secaucus, N.J.: Carol, 1999). The quoted excerpts are from pp. 19 and 22.

5. States mandating sex education and HIV-AIDS education appear in National Guidelines Task Force, *Guidelines for Comprehensive Sexuality Education: Kindergarten–12th Grade* (New York: SIECUS, 1991).

6. This quotation, which exemplifies the value of a comprehensive book for preadolescents, is from Ruth Westheimer, *Dr. Ruth Talks to Kids: Where You Came From, How Your Body Changes, and What Sex Is All About* (New York: Aladdin, 1998), p. 57.

7. For a discussion of changing Hispanic values in the bicultural environment, see B. H. Barkley and Enedian Salazar Mosher, "Sexuality and Hispanic Culture: Counseling with Children and Their Parents," *Journal of Sex Education and Therapy*, 1995, *21*, 255–267, and Miguel A. Perez and Helda L. Pinzon, "Sexual Communication Among Latino Adolescent Farm Workers: A Case Study," *American Journal of Health Studies*, 1997, *13*(2), 74–84.

8. For research on urban African American peer attitudes toward sex and pregnancy, see Bonita F. Stanton, Maureen Black, Linda Kaljee, and Izabel Ricardo, "Perceptions of Sexual Behavior Among Urban Early Adolescents: Translating Theory Through Focus Groups," *Journal of Early Adolescence*, 1993, *13*, 44–66.

6. Teaching Kids from Twelve to Seventeen

1. Regarding the theory of adolescent identity development, see Erikson, *Childhood and Society*, 2nd ed. rev., and Erik H. Erikson, *Identity, Youth, and Crisis* (New York: Norton, 1968).

2. Regarding various risk factors for early sexual activity, see Bonita F. Stanton and others, "Sexual Practices and Intentions Among Preadolescent and Early Adolescent Low-Income Urban African-Americans," *Pediatrics*, 1994, *93*, 966–974; Patricia East and Marianne E. Felice, "Sisters' and Girlfriends' Sexual and Childbearing Behavior: Effects on Early Adolescent Girls' Sexual Outcomes," *Journal of Marriage and the Family*, 1993, *55*, 963–964; Miller and others, "Pubertal Development"; Miller and others, "The Timing of Sexual Intercourse"; Whitbeck and others, "The Influence of Parental Support"; and Valois and others, "Number of Sexual Intercourse Partners."

3. This hypothesized model of adolescent decision making appeared in Lilly M. Langer and George J. Warheit, "The Pre-Adult Health Decision-Making Model: Linking Decision-Making Directedness/Orientation to Adolescent Health-Related Attitudes and Behaviors," *Adolescence*, 1992, *27*(109), 919–948.

4. For research on girls' first sexual intercourse, see Sharon Thompson, "Putting a Big Thing into a Little Hole: Teenage Girls' Accounts of Sexual

Initiation," *Journal of Sex Research*, 1990, *27*, 341–361. See also Sharon Thompson, *Going All the Way: Teenage Girls' Tales of Sex, Romance, and Pregnancy* (New York: Hill & Wang, 1995).

5. Two articles that deal with boys' reactions to intercourse and their sense of choice are Doreen A. Rosenthal, Susan M. Moore, and Irene Flynn, "Adolescent Self-Efficacy, Self-Esteem, and Sexual Risk-Taking," *Journal of Community and Applied Social Psychology*, 1991, *1*, 77–88, and Charlene Muehlenhard and Stephen W. Cook, "Men's Self-Reports of Unwanted Sexual Activity," *Journal of Sex Research*, 1988, *24*, 58–72.

6. Findings of satisfaction and other outcomes of first intercourse appeared in Woody and others, "Adolescent Non-Coital Sexual Activity."

7. This report on oral sex among young adolescents appeared in "Sexual Experimentation Takes Risky Turn Among Adolescents," reprinted from the *Washington Post* in the *Omaha World Herald*, July 15, 1999, p. 10.

About the Author

Jane DiVita Woody is professor of social work at the University of Nebraska at Omaha, where she has taught in the graduate program for twenty-five years. She holds a Ph.D. in English from Michigan State University and an M.S.W. from Western Michigan University. She is a clinical member and approved supervisor of the American Association for Marriage and Family Therapy and a certified sex therapist (American Association of Sex Educators, Counselors and Therapists).

Woody is the author of *Treating Sexual Distress: Integrative Systems Therapy* (Sage, 1992) and has published research and other articles on divorce, sex therapy, ethics, marriage and family therapy, and youth mentoring. She has also been a frequent presenter at professional conferences.

Index